Joint-Preserving Osteotomies for Malunited Foot & Ankle Fractures

Editor

STEFAN RAMMELT

FOOT AND ANKLE CLINICS

www.foot.theclinics.com

Consulting Editor
MARK S. MYERSON

March 2016 • Volume 21 • Number 1

ELSEVIER

1600 John F. Kennedy Boulevard • Suite 1800 • Philadelphia, Pennsylvania, 19103-2899

http://www.theclinics.com

FOOT AND ANKLE CLINICS Volume 21, Number 1
March 2016 ISSN 1083-7515, ISBN-13: 978-0-323-44400-2

Editor: Jennifer Flynn-Briggs
Developmental Editor: Meredith Clinton

Foot and Ankle Clinics (ISSN 1083-7515) is published quarterly by Elsevier, Inc., 360 Park Avenue South, New York, NY 10010-1710. Months of issue are March, June, September, and December. Periodicals postage paid at New York, NY, and additional mailing offices. Subscription price per year is $320.00 (US individuals), $466.00 (US institutions), $100.00 (US students), $360.00 (Canadian individuals), $560.00 (Canadian institutions), $215.00 (Canadian students), $460.00 (international individuals), $560.00 (international institutions), and $215.00 (international students). To receive student/resident rate, orders must be accompanied by name of affiliated institution, date of term, and the *signature* of program/residency coordinator on institution letterhead. Orders will be billed at individual rate until proof of status is received. Foreign air speed delivery is included in all *Clinics* subscription prices. All prices are subject to change without notice. **POSTMASTER:** Send address changes to *Foot and Ankle Clinics*, Elsevier Health Sciences Division, Subscription Customer Service, 3251 Riverport Lane, Maryland Heights, MO 63043. **Customer Service: 1-800-654-2452 (US and Canada). From outside of the United States and Canada, call 314-447-8871. Fax: 314-447-8029. E-mail: JournalsCustomerService-usa@ elsevier.com (for print support); JournalsOnlineSupport-usa@elsevier.com (for online support).**

Reprints. For copies of 100 or more, of articles in this publication, please contact the Commercial Reprints Department, Elsevier Inc., 360 Park Avenue South, New York, NY 10010-1710. Tel.: 212-633-3874; Fax: 212-633-3820; E-mail: reprints@elsevier.com.

Contributors

CONSULTING EDITOR

MARK S. MYERSON, MD
Director, Department of Orthopaedic Surgery, The Institute for Foot and Ankle Reconstruction, Mercy Hospital, Mercy Medical Center, Baltimore, Maryland

EDITOR

STEFAN RAMMELT, MD, PhD
Professor, Head of the Foot and Ankle Section, University Center for Orthopaedics and Traumatology, University Hospital Carl Gustav Carus at the TU Dresden, Dresden, Germany

AUTHORS

SHAFIC SAID AL-NAMMARI, MD, MSc(Oxon), FRCS(Tr&Orth)
International Foot and Ankle Fellow, The Institute for Foot and Ankle Reconstruction, Mercy Hospital, Mercy Medical Center, Baltimore, Maryland

ALEXEJ BARG, MD
Assistant Professor, Department of Orthopaedics, University of Utah, Salt Lake City, Utah

DANIEL BAUMFELD, MD
Master in Orthopaedics, Hospital Felicio Rocho, Belo Horizonte, Minas Gerais, Brazil; UFMG - Federal University of Minas Gerais - Foot and Ankle Surgery, Minas Gerais, Brazil

STEPHEN K. BENIRSCHKE, MD
Department of Orthopaedics and Sports Medicine, University of Washington, Seattle, Washington

BRIAN M. CAPOGNA, MD
Orthopaedic Surgery Resident Physician, Department of Orthopaedic Surgery, Hospital for Joint Diseases, New York University Langone Medical Center, New York, New York

MICHAEL CLARE, MD
University of South Florida Department of Orthopaedic Surgery, Florida Orthopaedic Institute, Tampa, Florida

KENNETH A. EGOL, MD
Professor, Vice Chair of Education, Department of Orthopaedic Surgery, Hospital for Joint Diseases, New York University Langone Medical Center, New York, New York

BEAT HINTERMANN, MD
Chairman and Associate Professor, Department of Orthopaedics and Trauma, Kantonsspital Baselland, Liestal, Switzerland

JOHN KETZ, MD
Department of Orthopaedic Surgery, University of Rochester, Rochester, New York

PATRICIA A. KRAMER, PhD
Department of Anthropology, University of Washington, Seattle, Washington

FABIAN KRAUSE, MD
Department of Orthopaedic Surgery, Inselspital, University of Berne, Berne, Switzerland

WOO-CHUN LEE, MD, PhD
Professor, Department of Orthopaedic Surgery, Seoul Foot and Ankle Center, Seoul Paik Hospital, Inje University, Seoul, South Korea

MARK S. MYERSON, MD
Director, Department of Orthopaedic Surgery, The Institute for Foot and Ankle Reconstruction, Mercy Hospital, Mercy Medical Center, Baltimore, Maryland

CAIO NERY, MD, PhD
Albert Einstein Hospital, Foot and Ankle Clinic, Hospital Israelita Albert Einstein, Morumbi; UNIFESP - Federal University of São Paulo - Foot and Ankle Surgery, São Paulo, Brazil

FLORIAN NICKISCH, MD
Associate Professor, Department of Orthopaedics, University of Utah, Salt Lake City, Utah

FERNANDO RADUAN, MD
Albert Einstein Hospital, Foot and Ankle Clinic, Hospital Israelita Albert Einstein, Morumbi; UNIFESP - Federal University of São Paulo - Foot and Ankle Surgery, São Paulo, Brazil

STEFAN RAMMELT, MD, PhD
Professor, Head of the Foot and Ankle Section, University Center for Orthopaedics and Traumatology, University Hospital Carl Gustav Carus at the TU Dresden, Dresden, Germany

ROY SANDERS, MD
Chairman, University of South Florida Department of Orthopaedic Surgery, Florida Orthopaedic Institute, Tampa, Florida

TIMO SCHMID, MD
Department of Orthopaedic Surgery, Inselspital, University of Berne, Berne, Switzerland

WOLFGANG SCHNEIDERS, MD, PhD
Professor, University Center for Orthopaedics and Traumatology, University Hospital Carl Gustav Carus at the TU Dresden, Dresden, Germany

THOMAS SUTER, MD
Attending Surgeon, Department of Orthopaedics and Trauma, Kantonsspital Baselland, Liestal, Switzerland

ANDREA VELJKOVIC, MD
Clinical Lecturer, University of Toronto, University of Health Network, Vancouver, British Columbia, Canada

DANIEL WEBER, MD
Department of Orthopaedics and Traumatology, St. Claraspital, Basel, Switzerland

MARTIN WEBER, MD
Professor, Department of Orthopaedics and Traumatology, Siloah AG, Gümligen, Switzerland

NICHOLAS J. WEGNER, MD
Fellow, Foot and Ankle Surgery, Department of Orthopaedics, University of Utah, Salt Lake City, Utah

YUN-FENG YANG, MD
Department of Orthopedics, Tongji Hospital, School of Medicine, Tongji University, Shanghai, China

GUANG-RONG YU, MD
Department of Orthopedics, Tongji Hospital, School of Medicine, Tongji University, Shanghai, China

MING-ZHU ZHANG, MD, PhD
Department of Orthopedics, Tongji Hospital, School of Medicine, Tongji University, Shanghai, China

HANS ZWIPP, MD, PhD
Professor Emeritus, Foot and Ankle Section, University Center for Orthopaedics and Traumatology, University Hospital Carl Gustav Carus at the TU Dresden, Dresden, Germany

Contents

Supramalleolar osteotomies of the tibia (SMOT) for posttraumatic distal tibial malalignment have shown to reduce pain, improve function and radiographic signs of osteoarthritis, and delay ankle arthrodesis or total joint replacement. The procedure also protects the articular cartilage from further degenerative processes by shifting and redistributing loads in the ankle joint. It is technically demanding and requires extensive preoperative planning. The type of osteotomy (opening vs closing wedge) does not influence the final outcome. However, based on the limited evidence, a grade I treatment recommendation has been given for supramalleolar osteotomies of the tibia to treat mild to moderate ankle arthritis in the presence of distal tibial malalignment.

Asymmetric ankle osteoarthritis (OA) is an increasingly recognized condition. It is imperative to differentiate between extraarticular and intraarticular deformity, and to address them appropriately. Any associated instability and multilevel deformity must be recognized and addressed. Patients with intraarticular varus or valgus asymmetric OA have poorer outcomes and higher rates of recurrence when treated with standard techniques targeted at correction with traditional supramalleolar or inframalleolar techniques. Plafondplasty aims to correct the deformity at its center of rotation and angulation and is associated with low rates of recurrence, substantial postoperative pain relief, functional improvement, and a possible slowing of the degenerative process.

The supramalleolar osteotomy has been reported to be a joint preserving surgery with good clinical outcome for asymmetric ankle osteoarthritis, especially varus ankle osteoarthritis. Conventional supramalleolar osteotomy of the tibia and fibula creates angulation and translation of the ankle joint without changing the width of the ankle mortise. Distal tibial oblique osteotomy improved the preoperative clinical and radiological parameters; however, mean talar tilt angle did not decrease. Assessment of the ankle arthritis in sagittal, axial, and coronal planes may be helpful to achieve a decrease of the talar tilt in ankle osteoarthritis.

posttraumatic talar malunion results in varus malalignment of the talar neck and can lead to painful overload of the lateral foot and substantial impairment of hindfoot function. Secondary procedures in patients with painful malunited talar neck fracture include salvage procedures and anatomic reconstruction procedures. Anatomic reconstruction of the talar neck is a reliable surgical treatment to regain function, decrease pain, and restore hindfoot alignment and range of motion.

Malunions and nonunions after central or peripheral fractures of the talar body frequently lead to pain and disability. In properly selected, compliant patients without symptomatic arthritis or total avascular necrosis leading to collapse of the talar dome, and sufficient bone stock, secondary anatomic reconstruction with osteotomy along the former fracture plane and preservation of the essential peritalar joints may lead to considerable functional improvement. Bone grafting is needed after resection of a fibrous pseudarthrosis, sclerotic, or necrotic bone. Malunions and nonunions of the lateral or posterior process are treated with excision of the malunited or loose fragments.

Intraarticular calcaneal fracture treatments that result in malalignment often require reconstructive surgery. Seven cases are used to demonstrate the intricacies of reconstructive case management. Reestablishment of calcaneal height, length, orientation, and position relative to the other tarsals is necessary to reestablish appropriate foot function. Inherent or acquired gastrocnemius equinus should be treated with recession to reduce destructive forces on the reconstruction.

Displaced tongue-type fractures of the calcaneus can lead to severe pain and disability if not treated appropriately. Failure to reduce articular displacement may require subtalar joint arthrodesis with subsequent loss of function. The subtalar joint is crucial for normal foot and ankle function. In selected cases, if the malunited joint is still in good condition, it is preserved by corrective osteotomy. A joint-preserving osteotomy with axial realignment is a treatment option for malunited tongue-type calcaneal fractures encountered early on, before the development of subtalar arthrosis in carefully selected patients.

The most effective way to treat calcaneal malunions is avoidance. With any articular fracture, progressive arthrosis and dysfunction are common. By restoring the anatomy initially through reduction, late reconstructive options become less complicated. Numerous studies have shown that restoration of the anatomic alignment either through percutaneous or open techniques is effective. In patients with no or minimal articular degeneration, extrarticular joint-sparing procedures can be performed. This represents a small select group who may benefit from simple osteotomy procedures with associated soft tissue reconstruction, if needed.

Treatment of malunion and nonunion at the Chopart joint aims at axial realignment of the midfoot to the hindfoot and restoration of the normal relationship of the lateral and medial columns of the foot. In carefully selected patients with intact cartilage, joint-preserving osteotomies are feasible at all 4 bony components of the Chopart joint to restore near-normal function. Priority should be given to the anatomic reconstruction of the talonavicular joint because it is essential for global foot function. Patients must be counseled about the risk of progressive arthritis or osteonecrosis necessitating late fusion.

Lisfranc fracture–dislocations are very serious and potentially disabling injuries. Unfortunately, they are often misdiagnosed. Multiplanar midfoot deformities that result from these fracture–dislocations are precursors of joint degeneration and significant functional disabilities. Anatomic reduction with different types of internal fixation is an efficient method to reconstruct midfoot alignment and stability. Joint-preserving reconstruction techniques emerge as a viable alternative to corrective fusion as they achieve stable joint realignment with preserved motion.

FOOT AND ANKLE CLINICS

RELATED INTEREST

Clinics in Podiatric Medicine and Surgery, July 2015 (Vol. 22, No. 3)
Foot and Ankle Osteotomies
Christopher F. Hyer, *Editor*
Available at: http://www.podiatric.theclinics.com

THE CLINICS ARE NOW AVAILABLE ONLINE!
Access your subscription at:
www.theclinics.com

Preface

Anatomical Reconstruction for Malunited Foot and Ankle Fractures

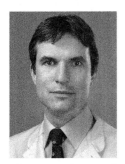

Stefan Rammelt, MD, PhD
Editor

Malunions and nonunions after foot and ankle fractures regularly result in painful deformities and severe functional restrictions in the affected patients. The mainstay of treatment for most of these conditions is a corrective fusion with the aim of reducing pain and achieving a stable, plantigrade foot. For most of the joints, there is no feasible prosthetic replacement option. Joint-sparing corrections aim at anatomic realignment of bones and joints in order to regain a maximum of foot function.

Since the classical works of B.G. Weber, realignment osteotomies at the ankle are widely used to correct malunited malleolar fractures, and favorable long-term results have been reported. Supramalleolar osteotomies are established for extra-articular malunions and deformities, and these techniques have been refined. Over recent years, joint-preserving corrections, including extra-articular and intra-articular osteotomies without fusion, have been increasingly used for virtually every bone of the foot starting with the talus, which is of utmost importance for global foot function.

The articles in this issue reiterate that proper patient selection is the key to success. Joint-preserving osteotomies may be considered in compliant patients with good bone and cartilage quality and without symptomatic arthritis at the time of presentation. Sometimes, the definite decision to save or fuse a joint will be made during corrective surgery, which has to be discussed with the patient in advance. On the other hand, performing a joint-sparing correction does not burn any bridges, and any necessary late fusion can be done as an in situ fusion in a well-aligned foot, which carries less risks than a corrective fusion in a malaligned foot.

I am extremely grateful that a formidable group of experienced foot and ankle surgeons from three continents agreed to contribute to this issue despite their notoriously

Foot Ankle Clin N Am 21 (2016) xiii–xiv
http://dx.doi.org/10.1016/j.fcl.2015.12.001
1083-7515/16/$ – see front matter © 2016 Published by Elsevier Inc.

foot.theclinics.com

full calendar. A special reference goes to my long-term mentor and surgical teacher, Hans Zwipp, MD, PhD, who profoundly influenced my approach to patients with malunions and nonunions at the foot and ankle. I sincerely hope that the readers will enjoy the articles of this issue as much as I did when reviewing them.

Stefan Rammelt, MD, PhD
University Center for Orthopaedics
and Traumatology
University Hospital Carl Gustav Carus at the TU Dresden
Fetscherstrasse 74
01307 Dresden
Germany

E-mail address:
strammelt@hotmail.com

Supramalleolar Osteotomies for Posttraumatic Malalignment of the Distal Tibia

 CrossMark

Fabian Krause, MD[a],*, Andrea Veljkovic, MD[b], Timo Schmid, MD[a]

KEYWORDS

• Distal tibia • Malalignment • Posttraumatic • Supramalleolar osteotomy

KEY POINTS

• Posttraumatic distal tibial malalignment can lead to asymmetric ankle arthritis in the long term.

• Supramalleolar osteotomy of the tibia (SMOT) in the management of posttraumatic malalignment of the distal tibia is designed to prevent the onset or delay the progression of asymmetric ankle arthritis.

• SMOT for posttraumatic distal tibial malalignment has shown to alleviate pain, improve function and radiographic signs of arthritis, and defer ankle arthrodesis or total ankle replacement.

• Generally, a significant improvement in functional and pain scores with good or excellent results in most patients is expected.

INTRODUCTION: NATURE OF THE PROBLEM

Posttraumatic distal tibial malalignment is usually sequelae of a previous physeal disturbance from a trauma in childhood, of a pilon fracture, or of a distal tibial shaft fracture. The malalignment comprises deformities in the coronal plane (varus and valgus), in the sagittal plane (flexion and extension), and malrotation either in isolation or in combination. Coronal and sagittal plane deformities change the mechanical axis, whereas altered load distribution may lead to asymmetric overload of the ankle's articular surface and arthritis in the long term. Trauma often additionally leads to direct cartilage shear or impaction and may attribute to ankle arthritis. Next to rotational

The authors have nothing to disclose.
[a] Department of Orthopaedic Surgery, Inselspital, University of Berne, Freiburgstrasse, Berne 3010, Switzerland; [b] University of Health Network, 1000–1200 Burrard Street, Vancouver, British Columbia V6Z2C7, Canada
* Corresponding author.
E-mail address: fabian.krause@insel.ch

fractures (37% of cases), recurrent sprains (15%), a single sprain (14%), and osteochondral lesions of the talus (5%), posttraumatic ankle arthritis has been shown to be attributable to a previous pilon fracture or a tibial shaft fracture in 9% each.[1] Previous studies have found an increased incidence of hindfoot disability and stiffness after malunited tibial fractures, which suggests that in the presence of tibial malunion realignment is advisable.[2,3]

The aim of supramalleolar osteotomies of the tibia (SMOT) in the management of posttraumatic malalignment of the distal tibia is to prevent the onset or delay the progression of asymmetric ankle arthritis. By transfer of the mechanical axis from the more arthritic part of the joint to an area with less affected articular cartilage, normalization of intra-articular load distribution is achieved.

Unless end-stage arthritis is already present, SMOT is an established treatment option particularly in younger adults, when other treatments, such as ankle arthrodesis or total ankle replacement, are less desirable or not yet indicated. Different techniques have been proposed, favoring either opening or closing wedge osteotomies in adults and mostly opening wedge osteotomies in children and adolescents. Alignment correction in ankle arthritis has been shown to reduce pain, improve function, decrease radiologic signs of arthritis, and therefore delay the need for fusion or joint replacement surgery.[4–10] Current evidence, however, is mainly based on level III or IV studies.

Biomechanics

Any deformity altering the load distribution across the tibiotalar joint may compromise the joint function and cartilage nutrition. However, there is no consensus in the literature considering the tolerable limits of distal tibial malalignment and the potential for development of ankle arthritis.[8] Biomechanical cadaver studies have shown that the contact surface area in the ankle joint is reduced up to 40% in the presence of malalignment.[11,12] Distal tibial malalignment substantially alters total tibiotalar contact area, contact shape, and contact location. Greater changes were detected with malalignment in the sagittal plane (40% for posterior and anterior angulation of 15°).[11] The subtalar joint plays an important role in retaining the talus in the correct alignment relative to the tibial axis. It acts as a torque transmitter and compensates tibial malalignment particularly in the coronal plane. Consequently, limited subtalar motion severely increases tibiotalar contact pressure changes from distal tibial malalignment.[12]

The decreased tibiotalar joint contact area leads to a pressure increase in the areas that remain loaded.[11] Circumscribed joint degeneration and cartilage wear add to the existing load concentration by an increasing talar tilt into the cartilage defect, thereby initiating the vicious circle of asymmetric ankle osteoarthritis.[7]

The SMOT aims for hindfoot realignment with transfer of the ankle back in line with the tibial weightbearing axis, normalization of intra-articular load distribution, and normalization of the direction of the triceps surae force vector.

Indications and Contraindication

The main indication for SMOT is asymmetric ankle arthritis caused by substantial malalignment in the coronal and less commonly in the sagittal plane. At least 50% of the ankle joint surface should be preserved. Further indications and contraindications are listed in **Table 1**.

Overcorrection

Most authors recommend an overcorrection of 3° to 5° in the coronal plane (tibial articular surface [TAS] angle 93°–95°),[7,10,11,13,14] whereas the amount of overcorrection is

Table 1 Indications and contraindications for SMOT	
Indications	Asymmetric ankle OA by supramalleolar and intra-articular valgus or varus malalignment
	Partially (>50%) preserved joint surface
	Osteochondral lesion of the medial or lateral ankle joint
	Supramalleolar and intra-articular malalignment in combination with TAR or AA
Absolute contraindications	End-stage degenerative changes of the complete tibiotalar joint
	Unmanageable hindfoot instability
	Acute or chronic infections
	Severe vascular or neurologic deficiency and neuropathic disorders (eg, Charcot arthropathy)
Relative contraindications	Noncompliance
	Patients older than 70 y and in poor general condition
	Substantially impaired bone quality of the distal tibia and/or talus (eg, patients on long-term steroid medication or with large subchondral cysts, severe osteoporosis, or rheumatic disease)
	Tobacco abuse

Abbreviations: AA, ankle arthrodesis; OA, osteoarthritis; TAR, total ankle replacement.

supposed to be adjusted to the severity of the ankle arthritis. Extensive overcorrection, however, may cause shear forces.[7] Takakura and colleagues[9] proposed a slight overcorrection based on photoelastic experiments in models and on their clinical experience. Most of their patients with fair results had undercorrection. Vichard and colleagues[13] suggested an overcorrection to more equally distribute the pressure in the ankle. However, Harstall and colleagues[15] planned their correction to neutral alignment of the tibial plafond only, not to decompensate the hindfoot into hypervalgus and to prevent creating a deformity that could compromise the results of a total ankle replacement later on. The favorable effect of the osteotomy could still be obtained.

Concomitant Procedures

Most orthopedic surgeons would rather reconstruct lateral and medial ligaments in pre-existing hindfoot instability (**Table 2**). However, there is clinical evidence that even without ligament reconstruction lateral hindfoot stability is consistently regained if an appropriate bony realignment is achieved.[10,11,16]

Table 2 Common concomitant procedure to restore full neutral alignment in cases of advanced ankle arthritis		
Malalignment	Soft Tissue Procedures	Bony Procedures
Varus	Deltoid release, repair or reconstruction of lateral ligaments	Lateralizing calcaneal osteotomy, plafond-plasty, fibula valgus osteotomy
Valgus	Repair or reconstruction of deltoid, spring ligament and posterior tibial tendon, release of lateral ligaments	Medializing calcaneal osteotomy, medial malleolus varus osteotomy

In case of ongoing talar tilt after the SMOT caused by an inadequate length of the fibula, or if the talus does not follow the medial malleolus because of ligamentous restriction, the fibula is osteotomized and the position and length of the fibula adjusted. A neutral alignment within the ankle joint is crucial for appropriate results. When a residual talar varus tilt is observed, a shortening and valgus osteotomy is performed. When a valgus talar tilt persists a varus osteotomy of the fibula is done in many cases. In severe malalignments, an additional lateralizing or medializing calcaneal osteotomy should be considered to attain full realignment.

Lateral-Closing Versus Medial-Opening Supramalleolar Osteotomies of the Tibia

The decision between the lateral or medial approach is mainly based on the surgeon's preference and the amount of correction needed. In extensive medial-opening wedge osteotomies, the fibula may restrict the amount of correction possible, even with a fibula osteotomy. Therefore, large deformities greater than 10° are better corrected through a lateral-closing SMOT.[15]

Advantages of the lateral-closing SMOT are an easy fixation, no bone graft requirement, reliable and rapid bone healing because of an inherent stability and a large osteotomy contact area, and no medial joint overload. The disadvantages are more soft tissue dissection with the additional fibular osteotomy and fixation, a possible weakening of the peroneals, and a possible leg shortening in large corrections.[15] However, lateral hindfoot instability and a noticeable leg length discrepancy after lateral-closing SMOT is not reported in the current literature.[15]

Medial-opening wedge osteotomies have the advantages of using a simple approach, ease of bone cuts, and no resultant leg shortening. Potential disadvantages are graft morbidity, failure of graft incorporation, a higher rate of delayed and nonunion of the osteotomy (5%–25%), necessity for greater fixation strength, and increase in the medial joint load by tensioning of the extrinsic medial tendons. Posttraumatic medial soft tissue tightness may cause additional tension on the neurovascular structures and tightening of the posterior tibial tendon in the varus malalignment. Often the fibula osteotomy is an additional operative step in larger corrections that requires a second approach.

SURGICAL TECHNIQUE FOR LATERAL-CLOSING SUPRAMALLEOLAR OSTEOTOMIES OF THE TIBIA
Preoperative Planning

Preoperative planning is an important part of this surgery. The planning of posttraumatic distal tibial malalignment follows the same rules as the planning of congenital distal tibial varus and valgus deformities.[15] The center of rotation and angulation (CORA) is analyzed on full-length weightbearing anteroposterior and lateral radiographs of the ankle and lower leg.[17,18] However, even when the CORA is proximal to the supramalleolar osteotomy level (ie, in the distal two-thirds of the tibial diaphysis), the osteotomy is in most cases preferably placed in the tibial metaphysis for better bone healing.[19,20] In addition, whole leg radiographs should be taken to assess osseous deformities of the lower extremity, particularly around the knee joint. In cases of multilevel injuries, a rotational computed tomography scan is advised to gather the whole extent of the malalignment.

To evaluate the coronal plane deformity, the TAS angle (norm: 0°–3° varus) is measured on the full-length tibial shaft radiographs in the coronal plane (**Fig. 1**A).[21,22] The tibiotalar angle (norm: 0°–2.5° varus tilt) describes the tilt of the talus within the ankle mortise (**Fig. 1**B). The tibial lateral surface angle (norm: 9°–10° anteriorly open) assesses

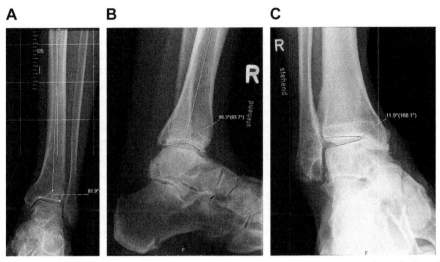

Fig. 1. Electronic measurement (picture archiving and communication system [PACS], digital images) of the (*A*) TAS (norm: 0°–3° varus), (*B*) the tibiotalar angle (norm: 0°–2.5° varus tilt), and (*C*) the tibial lateral surface angle (norm: 9°–10° anteriorly open). (*Data from* Mangone PG. Distal tibial osteotomies for the treatment of foot and ankle disorders. Foot Ankle Clin 2001;6:583–97; and Warnock KM, Johnson BD, Wright JB, et al. Calculation of the opening wedge for a low tibial osteotomy. Foot Ankle Int 2004;25:778–82.)

the flexion and extension deformity in the sagittal plane (**Fig. 1**C).[21,22] Ideally the normal TAS and tibial lateral surface angles can be compared with radiographs of the healthy contralateral limb. The degree of the arthritic changes in the ankle joint is classified on preoperative radiographs using the scale described by Katsui and colleagues[21] (**Table 3**).

To assess the severity of cartilage damage in the affected part and the cartilage quality in the unaffected part in cases of asymmetric ankle arthritis, MRI and single-photon emission computed tomography/computed tomography complete imaging options. If still in doubt whether the SMOT is indicated, a diagnostic ankle arthroscopy in advance as a second procedure or directly ahead of joint surgery is recommended.

The size of the correction wedge to be removed or opened is determined by drawing the desired correction angle on the preoperative radiographs and measuring the length of the wedge's base on a template while taking magnification into account,

Table 3
Classification of the degree of the arthritic changes in the ankle joint according to Takakura

Arthritis Grade	Radiographic Findings
Stage 1	No narrowing of the joint space but evidence of subchondral bone sclerosis and formation of osteophytes
Stage 2	Narrowing of the joint space medially or laterally
Stage 3	Obliteration of the medial or lateral joint space and contact between adjacent subchondral bone
Stage 4	Complete obliteration of the joint space with bone-to-bone contact

From Katsui T, Takakura Y, Kitada C, et al. Roentgenographic analysis for osteoarthrosis of the ankle joint. J Jpn Soc Surg Foot 1980;1:52–7.

or nowadays commonly electronically (PACS, digital images). The height of the wedge (H) to be removed can also be calculated using the formula $tan\,! = H/W$ (! = axial angle, H = wedge height, W = tibial width).[23]

If the deformity is in both the coronal and sagittal planes, a biplanar wedge modification is necessary to correct the deformity. If the talus is anteriorly extruded out of the mortise, the correction is conducted in a biplanar fashion (eg, additional anterior opening or posterior closing wedge, to improve talar coverage in the sagittal plane).[4] However, it has to taken into account that this osteotomy reduces ankle dorsiflexion. Depending on the severity of present asymmetric arthritis, an overcorrection up to 5° is recommended. In cases of advanced arthritis including a talar tilt within the ankle mortise, indicating cartilage or bony erosion, concomitant procedures may be required to restore full neutral alignment.

Preparation and Patient Positioning

The patients are prepared and draped in a standard way. In the lateral position, the leg with a thigh tourniquet on is placed on a tunnel-like bolster. A radiolucent operating table is required for use of intraoperative fluoroscopy.

Surgical Approach

Along the posterior aspect of the fibula, a 10- to 12-cm longitudinal skin incision is made. The fibula is dissected anteriorly cautiously sparing the periosteum. Without violating the perforator vessels from the fibular artery that runs posterior to the interosseous membrane until it penetrates the membrane from 3 to 5 cm above the syndesmosis, the interosseous membrane is exposed. For the exposure of the anterior aspect of the tibia, all anterior soft tissues are elevated, and a Hohmann retractor is securely positioned over the anterior tibial ridge to protect the extensor tendons and the anterior neurovascular bundle (**Fig. 2A**).

Then the peroneal fascia is opened along the posterolateral edge of the fibula and the peroneal tendons are retracted posteriorly for the posterior dissection. The fibers

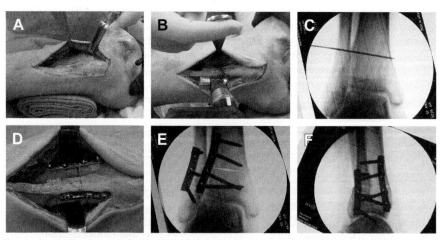

Fig. 2. (A–F) The lateral-closing SMOT. (A) Exposure of the distal tibia and fibula from lateral. (B, C) The osteostomy is marked with Kirschner wires under fluoroscopic guidance, and the cut following the guidewires is performed using an oscillating saw. (D) The SMOT is closed cautiously and fixed by 3.5-mm one-third tubular plates for the tibia and fibula. (E, F) Intraoperative fluoroscopic images of the fixation.

of the long flexor hallucis muscle originating from the posteromedial fibula are detached without violating the peroneal vessels running directly underneath the tenuous deep fascia. The muscle belly is bluntly elevated from the interosseous membrane and the posterior tibia until a Hohmann retractor can cautiously be placed to protect particularly the posterior tibial tendon.

Surgical Procedure

Step one
Three centimeters proximal to the ankle joint line a 1.6-mm Kirschner wire is drilled into the fibula and tibia from lateral to medial and rectangular to the tibial axis in both planes under fluoroscopic guidance. A second 1.6-mm Kirschner wire is placed in the same coronal plane but proximally, convergent, and distant to the first wire as measured preoperatively on the radiographs. The wires mark the desired bony wedge to be removed for the preoperatively calculated amount of correction. The wire tips should reach but not perforate the medial tibial cortex.

Step two
The depth of the Kirschner wires within the bone is measured and the first incomplete osteotomy is stopped 5 mm short of the medial cortex using a wide calibrated saw blade. Continuous water irrigation reduces thermal damage during the cutting process. The osteotomy follows the guidewires in a straight line, along the guidewire, considering the fibula and tibia as one bone (**Fig. 2**B, C). In the sagittal plane, the saw blade must be perpendicular to the tibial shaft. Under fluoroscopic guidance the second incomplete cut is directed to intersect the first cut just lateral to the medial tibial cortex. To facilitate orientation and ensure that the second cut is made in the same coronal plane, a saw blade is inserted half way into the first cut. An unintentional deviation in the coronal plane leads to an extension or flexion deformity. The lateral-based wedge is cautiously freed and removed without breaking the medial tibial hinge. For a controlled closure of the osteotomy the medial cortex should be weakened by several drill holes and a small osteotome.

Step three
The fixation of the osteotomy is achieved with two short 2.7-mm dynamic compression or 3.5-mm one-third tubular plates (**Fig. 2**D–E). They are positioned anterolateral on the tibia and posterolateral on the fibula for a stabile tension-band fixation technique and eccentrically drilled plate holes for compression of the osteotomy.

Step four
Appropriate correction and implant positioning and absence of medial hinge distraction are verified by fluoroscopy. A broken hinge has to be fixed by a medial plate to enhance stability and avoid delayed or nonunion. The wound is closed in two layers after irrigation and over a suction drain if required.

Immediate Postoperative Care

After the wound is closed, a split below-knee plaster of Paris or cast is applied and the leg is continuously kept elevated in bed. Once the wound is dry, the patient is mobilized and discharged but kept nonweightbearing in a closed below-knee cast. All patients receive thromboprophylaxis with subcutaneous low-molecular-weight heparin or oral medication, such as rivaroxaban, starting 12 hours preoperatively and continuing daily for 6 to 8 weeks postoperatively.

Rehabilitation and Recovery

The patients are seen depending on age, smoking and diabetes status, and intraoperatively achieved quality of fixation after 3 to 4 weeks in the outpatient clinic for a cast change and nonweightbearing anteroposterior and lateral radiographs of the ankle. Young and healthy patients are seen after 3 weeks, because an immobilization of a total of 6 weeks is usually sufficient. If wound and bone healing show appropriate progress, 10 to 20 kg partial weightbearing is permitted for another 3 to 4 weeks. In the second outpatient clinic visit the osteotomy is usually seen to be sufficiently stable to allow progress to full weightbearing without further casting. Ambulatory physiotherapy including extending active and passive ankle motion, stretching and strengthening of the lower leg musculature, and proprioceptive exercises is started.

In patients with persistent swelling, we recommend the use of compression stockings. Standard further visits are scheduled 3 and 12 months postoperatively. Sports and recreational activities are resumed 3 to 4 months postoperatively.

SURGICAL TECHNIQUE FOR MEDIAL-OPENING SUPRAMALLEOLAR OSTEOTOMIES OF THE TIBIA

The medial-opening wedge SMOT is indicated in cases with a varus deformity less than 10°.

Preoperative Planning

The preoperative planning follows the same rules as for lateral-closing SMOT, whereas it is not the size of the wedge that is calculated but the height of the gap to be opened for realignment.

Preparation and Patient Positioning

The patients are operated in the supine position. Preparation and patient positioning are as for lateral-closing SMOT.

Surgical Approach

An 8- to 10-cm medial longitudinal incision is centered over the distal tibia and medial malleolus. Care is taken not to injure the saphenous nerve and vein. To protect the anterior and posteromedial neurovascular bundles and tendons, the soft tissues are reflected as one using two Hohmann retractors.

Surgical Procedure

Step one
Three centimeters proximal to the ankle joint line one or two 1.6-mm Kirschner wires are drilled into the tibia from medial to lateral and rectangular to the tibial axis in both planes under fluoroscopic guidance (**Fig. 3**A).

Step two
The osteotomy is performed using a wide saw blade to avoid an uneven osteotomy surface, which would impair bone healing (**Fig. 3**B). Continuous water irrigation reduces thermal damage during the cutting process. The depth of the Kirschner wires in bone is measured and the incomplete osteotomy is stopped 5 mm short of the lateral cortex to enhance the intrinsic stability of the osteotomy.

Step three
For a controlled opening of the osteotomy the lateral tibial cortex should be weakened by several drill holes and a small osteotome. For the opening of the

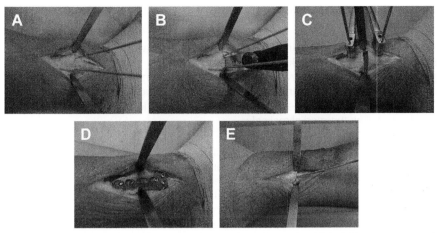

Fig. 3. (A–E) The medial opening SMOT in a cadaver lower leg. (A, B) The osteostomy is marked with Kirschner wires under fluoroscopic guidance, and the cut following the guidewires is performed using an oscillating saw. (C) For the opening of the osteotomy, a Kirschner wire spreader is used, and the gap is packed with a unicortical structural autograft. (D) The osteotomy is fixed with an upside down T-shaped 3.5-mm locking compression plate. (E) Oblique osteotomy of the fibula fixed with a 3.5-mm one-third tubular plate.

osteotomy, a laminar spreader or Kirschner wire spreader can be used (**Fig. 3**C). The gap is packed by cancellous or unicortical structural autograft harvested from the ipsilateral iliac crest bone or allograft. Cancellous bone graft is preferred for smaller osteotomies and good fixation quality of the osteotomy, whereas cases with large correction and poor bony purchase may benefit from structural bone graft. Allograft avoids morbidity from harvesting, speeds up surgery, but is more expensive. The osteotomy is fixed with an upside down T-shaped 3.5-mm locking compression plate (**Fig. 3**D).

Step four
Appropriate correction and implant positioning and absence of lateral hinge distraction are verified by fluoroscopy. A broken hinge has to be fixed by a lateral tibial plate to improve stability and avoid delayed or nonunion. The wound is closed in two layers after irrigation and over a suction drain if required.

Step five
A valgus (and rarely shortening) osteotomy of the fibula is simultaneously performed when needed in large corrections or when the talus remains tilted in the cartilage defect after the SMOT. The osteotomy is done oblique to increase the bony surface for better healing (**Fig. 3**E). It is secured with a 3.5-mm one-third tubular plate.

Immediate Postoperative Care

This is performed as with lateral-closing SMOT.

Rehabilitation and Recovery

These are performed as with lateral-closing SMOT.

SURGICAL TECHNIQUE FOR MEDIAL-CLOSING SUPRAMALLEOLAR OSTEOTOMIES OF THE TIBIA

Preparation, patient positioning, and surgical approach are the same as for medial-opening SMOT. Because closing osteotomies provide superior inherent stability, appropriate fixation is achieved with two short 2.7-mm dynamic compression or two 3.5-mm one-third tubular plates applied in an angle of about 60° to each other. Typically, an osteotomy of the fibula is needed to restore joint congruency or to allow the talus to follow the medial malleolus.

Alternative Surgical Techniques

Lee and colleagues[6] described an oblique osteotomy plane for the SMOT, which was placed at the apex of the syndesmosis. They stated that this SMOT minimizes the adverse effect of mortise distortion and enhanced osteotomy site stability because of the presence of an intact fibula.

In severe and/or multiplanar deformities and in deformities that are corrected at a level other than the CORA a dome-shaped or "pendulum" osteotomy reduces the translation of the osteotomized distal tibia that inevitably accompanies large corrections. In the "pendulum" osteotomy a wedge of half of the tibial width representing half of the desired correction is removed and installed on the contralateral side (**Fig. 4**).

Complications

Intraoperative complications are injuries of neurovascular structures and tendons. Exact anatomic knowledge of surgical approaches is prerequisite. Superficial wound healing problems and infections may be resolved by antibiotics, deeper problems

A　　　　　**B**　　　　　　**C**

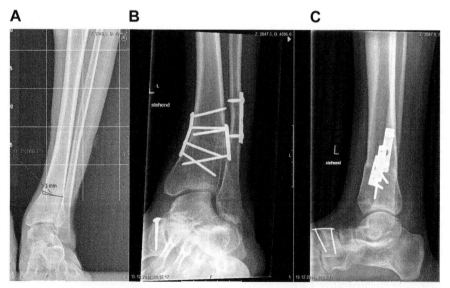

Fig. 4. (A–C) Radiographs of a 17-year-old boy with an unspecific dysmorphia of the lower legs. The 22° valgus malalignment in the coronal plane was corrected by a "pendulum" osteotomy to minimize translation of the distal tibia. An 11° wedge of half of the tibia was removed from the medial tibia and installed into the completely osteotomized lateral tibia. Fixation was achieved with two 2.7-mm dynamic compression plates. For unlimited correction the fibula was also osteotomized and fixed with a 3.5-mm one-third tubular plate.

Table 4
Outcome after SMOT

Author	LOE	Patients	Average Follow-up (y)	SMOT Type	Complications	Outcome
Takakura et al,[9] 1995	IV	18	6.9	Medial-opening	Delayed union (4), undercorrection (2)	Excellent (6), good (9), fair (3), no poor
Takakura et al,[20] 1998	IV	9	7.3	Medial-opening	Delayed union (2), decreased ROM (6), persistent medial pain (2)	Takakura score 100 pts. score, 69 ≥ 87
Cheng et al,[14] 2001	IV	18	4	Medial-opening with oblique fibula	Late infection (1), delayed union (2)	Own 100 pts. score, 50 ≥ 88
Stamatis et al,[8] 2003	IV	12 (13 ankles)	2.8	Medial-closing (7), medial-opening (6)	Delayed union (1), decreased ROM (3), superficial infection (1)	AOFAS, 54 ≥ 87
Tanaka et al,[10] 2006	IV	25 (26 ankles)	8.3	Anteromedial-opening	Delayed union (6), OA progression requiring AA (2) and conservative treatment (2)	Takakura score 100 pts. score, 51 ≥ 79
Harstall et al,[15] 2007	IV	9	4.7	Lateral-closing	OA progression requiring AA (1)	AOFAS, 48 ≥ 74
Pagenstert et al,[26] 2008	II	35	5	Medial-closing (18), medial-opening (7), lateral-closing (4)	OA progression requiring TAR (3), nonunion (2), recurrent deformity (2), wound healing problems (2), implant removal (7)	AOFAS, 39 ≥ 85
Neumann et al,[27] 2007	IV	27	2.5	Lateral-closing	OA progression requiring TAR (3) or ankle arthrodesis (3)	21 very satisfied
Knupp et al,[5] 2011	II	92 (94 ankles)	3.6	Medial-closing (61), lateral-closing or medial-opening (33)	Superficial wound healing problems (5), deep infection (1), anterior tibial tendon laceration (1), painful neuroma of the saphenous nerve (2), OA progression requiring TAR (9) or ankle arthrodesis (1)	AOFAS, 56 ≥ 73
Lee et al,[6] 2011	IV	16	2.3	Oblique medial-opening without fibular OT	None	AOFAS, 62 ≥ 82

Abbreviations: AA, ankle arthrodesis; AOFAS, American Orthopaedic Foot and Ankle Society; LOE, level of evidence; OA, osteoarthritis; OT, osteotomy; pts, patients; ROM, range of motion; TAR, total ankle replacement.

rather by surgical debridement and irrigation in addition. Painful neuromas may occur when nerves are injured. An inappropriate surgical technique may cause malunion or nonunion at the osteotomy site in the short or medium term. For instance, compromising the opposite cortex, nonanatomic reduction, secondary displacement of the osteotomy (eg, caused by noncompliance) during the postoperative rehabilitation, or inappropriate fixation leading to hardware breakage may lead to failure. The patients should also be aware that a joint-sacrificing operation, ankle arthrodesis, or arthroplasty might be inevitable later on.

CLINICAL RESULTS IN THE LITERATURE

Generally, a substantial improvement in functional and pain scores with good or excellent results in most patients is expected after SMOT. The reported average improvement in the American Orthopaedic Foot and Ankle Society ankle hindfoot score is 33 points of a total of 100. The osteotomies for varus ankle arthritis have been shown to delay the originally planned ankle arthrodesis or total ankle replacement in more than 90% of patients.[7] However, only the minority of patients is able to perform sports and recreational activities as desired. Any activities that cause pain and swelling of the joint should be discouraged because of the higher risk for revision. The major risk factors for early failures after SMOT are advanced stages of ankle arthritis, ankle joint instability, and joint incongruency.[14] Particularly, the combination of a distal tibia varus alignment with varus talar tilt and degenerative changes located in the medial gutter has led to inferior outcome, and a plafond plasty (eg, an intraarticular osteotomy) has been recommended to restore the joint geometry in these cases.[7,24] Further clinical results are listed in **Table 4**.

SUMMARY

SMOT for posttraumatic distal tibial malalignment has shown to reduce pain, improve function and radiographic signs of osteoarthritis, and delay ankle arthrodesis or total joint replacement. The procedure also protects the articular cartilage from further degenerative processes by shifting and redistributing loads in the ankle joint. It is technically demanding and requires extensive preoperative planning. The type of osteotomy (opening vs closing wedge) does not influence the final outcome. However, based on the limited evidence, a grade I (insufficient evidence) treatment recommendation has been given for SMOT to treat mild to moderate ankle arthritis in the presence of distal tibial malalignment malalignment.[25]

REFERENCES

1. Saltzman CL, Salomon ML, Blanchard GM, et al. Epidemiology of ankle arthritis: report of a consecutive series of 639 patients from a tertiary orthopaedic center. Iowa Orthop J 2005;25:44–6.
2. McMaster M. Disability of the hindfoot after fracture of the tibial shaft. J Bone Joint Surg 1976;58B:90–3.
3. Merriam WF, Porter KM. Hindfoot disability after a tibial shaft fracture treated by internal fixation. J Bone Joint Surg 1983;65B:326–8.
4. Knupp M, Hintermann B. Treatment of asymmetric arthritis of the ankle joint with supramalleolar osteotomies. Foot Ankle Int 2012;33:250–2.
5. Knupp M, Stufkens SA, Bolliger L, et al. Classification and treatment of supramalleolar deformities. Foot Ankle Int 2011;32:1023–31.

6. Lee WC, Moon JS, Lee K, et al. Indications for supramalleolar osteotomy in patients with ankle osteoarthritis and varus deformity. J Bone Joint Surg Am 2011; 93:1243–8.
7. Pagensteert GI, Hintermann B, Barg A, et al. Realignment surgery as alternative treatment of varus and valgus ankle osteoarthritis. Clin Orthop Rel Res 2007;462: 156–68.
8. Stamatis ED, Cooper PS, Myerson MS. Supramalleolar osteotomy for the treatment of distal tibial angualr deformities and arthritis of the ankle joint. Foot Ankle Int 2003;24:754–64.
9. Takakura Y, Tanaka Y, Kumai T, et al. Low tibial osteotomy for osteoarthritis of the ankle. J Bone Joint Surg Br 1995;77:50–4.
10. Tanaka Y, Takakura Y, Hayashi K, et al. Low tibial osteotomy for varus-type osteoarthritis of the ankle. J Bone Joint Surg Br 2006;88:909–13.
11. Tarr RR, Resnick CT, Wagner KS, et al. Changes in tibiotalar joint contact areas following experimentally induced tibial angular deformities. Clin Orthop 1985; 199:72–80.
12. Ting AJ, Tarr RR, Sarmiento A, et al. The role of subtalar motion and ankle contact pressure changes from angular deformities of the tibia. Foot Ankle 1987;7:290–9.
13. Vichard P, Gagneux E, Garbuio P, et al. Additional supra-mallleolar osteotomy. Rev Chir Orthop Reparatrice Appar Mot 1996;82:63–9.
14. Cheng Y-M, Huang P-J, Hong S-H, et al. Low tibial osteotomy for moderate ankle arthritis. Arch Orthop Trauma Surg 2001;121:355–8.
15. Harstall R, Lehmann O, Krause F, et al. Supramalleolar lateral-closing wedge osteotomy for the treatment of varus ankle arthrosis. Foot Ankle Int 2007;28: 542–8.
16. Krause F, Henning J, Pfander G, et al. Cavovarus foot realignment to treat anteromedial ankle arthrosis. Foot Ankle Int 2013;34:54–64.
17. Paley D, Herzenberg JE. Applications of external fixation to foot and ankle reconstruction. In: Myerson MS, editor. Foot and ankle disorders. Philadelphia: WB Saunders; 2000. p. 1135–88.
18. Paley D, Herzenberg JE, Tetsworth K, et al. Deformity planning for frontal and sagittal plane corrective osteotomies. Orthop Clin North Am 1994;25:425–65.
19. Graehl PM, Hersh MR, Heckman JD. Supramalleolar osteotomy for the treatment of symptomatic tibial malunion. J Orthop Trauma 1987;1:281–92.
20. Takakura Y, Takaoka T, Tanaka Y, et al. Results of opening-wedge osteotomy for the treatment of a post-traumatic varus deformity of the ankle. J Bone Joint Surg Am 1998;80:213–8.
21. Katsui T, Takakura Y, Kitada C, et al. Roentgenographic analysis for osteoarthrosis of the ankle joint. J Jpn Soc Surg Foot 1980;1:52–7.
22. Mangone PG. Distal tibial osteotomies for the treatment of foot and ankle disorders. Foot Ankle Clin 2001;6:583–97.
23. Warnock KM, Johnson BD, Wright JB, et al. Calculation of the opening wedge for a low tibial osteotomy. Foot Ankle Int 2004;25:778–82.
24. Mann HA, Myerson M, Filippi J. Results of medial opening wedge supramalleolar osteotomy (plafond plasty) for the treatment of intraarticular varus ankle arthritis and ankle instability. Presented at the 26th Annual Summer Meeting of the American Orthopaedic Foot and Ankle Society. Maryland, July 9, 2010.
25. Labib SA, Raikin SM, Lau JT, et al. Joint preservation procedures for ankle arthritis. Foot Ankle Int 2013;34:1040–7.

26. Pagenstert G, Leumann A, Hintermann B, et al. Sports and recreation activity of varus and valgus ankle osteoarthritis before and after realignment surgery. Foot Ankle Int 2008;29:985–93.
27. Neumann HW, Lieske S, Schenk K. Supramalleolar, subtractive valgus osteotomy of the tibia in the management of ankle joint degeneration with varus deformity. Oper Orthop Traumatol 2007;19:511–26.

The Use of Tibial Osteotomy (Ankle Plafondplasty) for Joint Preservation of Ankle Deformity and Early Arthritis

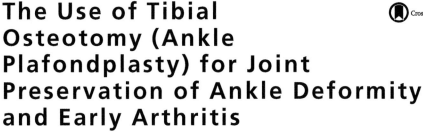 CrossMark

Shafic Said Al-Nammari, MD, MSc(Oxon), FRCS(Tr&Orth)*,
Mark S. Myerson, MD

KEYWORDS

- Tibia osteotomy • Ankle arthritis • Asymmetric • Varus ankle • Valgus ankle
- Plafondplasty

KEY POINTS

- Asymmetric ankle osteoarthritis (OA) is an increasingly recognized condition and it is imperative to differentiate between extraarticular and intraarticular deformity and to address these appropriately.
- Associated instability and multilevel deformity must be recognized and addressed.
- Patients with intraarticular varus or valgus asymmetric OA have poorer outcomes and higher rates of recurrence when treated with standard extraarticular supramalleolar and inframalleolar osteotomies.
- Plafondplasty is an intraarticular osteotomy and aims to correct the deformity at its center of rotation and angulation.

INTRODUCTION

The prevalence of ankle osteoarthritis (OA) is 1% to 4%[1] with an incidence of 48 per 100,000 per annum.[2] Owing to the advancing age of the population, this is set to increase significantly.[3,4] Although the incidence of ankle OA remains far lower than that in the hip or knee, its clinical importance should not be underestimated. It has been demonstrated that the physical and mental disability associated with end-stage ankle OA is at least as severe as that of end stage OA affecting the hip.[5]

In contrast with the hip and knee, the incidence of primary OA in the ankle is low with secondary OA being far more common.[1,6] Trauma remains the single most common

The authors have nothing to disclose.
The Institute for Foot & Ankle Reconstruction, Mercy Hospital, Mercy Medical Center, 301 St Paul Place, Baltimore, MD 21202, USA
* Corresponding author.
E-mail address: shafic2@hotmail.com

Foot Ankle Clin N Am 21 (2016) 15–26
http://dx.doi.org/10.1016/j.fcl.2015.09.009
1083-7515/16/$ – see front matter © 2016 Elsevier Inc. All rights reserved.

foot.theclinics.com

cause of secondary ankle OA accounting for approximately 80%.[6,7] The most common cause of posttraumatic ankle OA is a fracture of the ankle but chronic ankle instability is an increasingly recognized cause.[8,9] In contrast with primary OA, which affects the joint symmetrically, posttraumatic ankle OA frequently affects the joint asymmetrically resulting in a valgus or varus deformity of the ankle[10] (**Box 1**).

Ankles with pathologic valgus and varus deformities suffer from lateral and medial joint overload, respectively, with associated subsequent lateral or medial tibiotalar joint degeneration. This in turn causes further lateral/medial load shift resulting in a vicious cycle of ever-increasing mechanical malalignment.[11] In many of these cases of asymmetrical ankle OA, the presenting patients are comparatively young making joint-sacrificing procedures such as total ankle replacement or ankle arthrodesis less attractive treatment options.[1] In these cases, joint-preserving realignment surgery to unload the affected area and attempt to normalize joint biomechanics is particularly attractive. Without realignment, asymmetric ankle OA progresses to generalized end-stage ankle OA.[12,13] Traditionally, these have been extraarticular. The senior author (M.S.M.) had noted that there was a group of patients where the deformity was in fact truly intraarticular. In these cases, chronic varus and valgus stresses result in depression of the medial or lateral tibial plafond respectively. Despite the ability of these extraarticular osteotomies to realign the mechanical axis, they did not address the intraarticular pathology and over time there was a tendency for the talus to fall back into the depression and the deformity to recur.

Substantial ankle malalignment is common in ankles with end-stage OA. The ability of the foot and ankle to tolerate deformity above or at the level of the ankle depends, to a significant extent, on the flexibility of the foot to secondarily accommodate and compensate for this deformity. With a proximal varus or valgus deformity, the subtalar joint must evert or invert to maintain a plantigrade foot. The subtalar joint often compensates for the malaligned ankle in static weight bearing[14] and is able to accommodate more valgus than varus.[12,14] Owing to this ability of the subtalar joint to better accommodate valgus and the association with instability,[9] asymmetric varus OA is more common than asymmetric valgus OA of the ankle.[1,15] However, regardless of

---

Box 1
Etiology of ankle asymmetric osteoarthritis

Valgus

Intraarticular fracture: shortened externally rotated fibula/valgus impacted plafond

Chronic medial instability

Posterior tibial tendon dysfunction grade IV

Tarsal coalition

Pes planovalgus

Primary

Varus

Intraarticular fracture: Varus impacted plafond

Chronic lateral instability

Cavovarus deformity

Primary

the ability of the subtalar joint to compensate for varus or valgus deformity, the mechanics of the ankle joint remain abnormal and, ultimately, irreversible articular damage occurs.

To date, only short- to mid-term results of realignment surgery are available. These results are promising, with substantial improvements in pain, functional outcomes, and patient satisfaction reported for these procedure.[16–20] The aim of these surgeries is to realign the mechanical axis and alter the load transfer through the joint to the unaffected compartment. In general, these procedures aim to alter the alignment either above or below the level of the ankle joint. Above the ankle joint, a variety of opening and closing wedge supramalleolar osteotomies have been reported with varied success.[17,21–24] Below the ankle joint, calcaneal osteotomy, subtalar arthrodesis, first tarsometatarsal joint arthrodesis, medial deltoid release or reconstruction, and lateral reconstruction have all been trialed in an effort to straighten and balance the foot and ankle. Failure of all of these techniques is more likely to occur in those cases with medial or lateral intraarticular defects, because they are not addressed directly. With chronic varus and valgus stress, there can be erosion of the medial and lateral distal tibia, respectively. The talus falls into this defect resulting in intraarticular ankle varus or valgus. Furthermore, in varus cases the medial malleolus can erode and become inclined medially instead of vertical, which further adds to the likelihood of recurrent deformity.

The senior author (M.S.M.) has trialed the various supramalleolar and inframalleolar procedures listed to attempt joint preservation in these cases. In keeping with other authors experiences, this author noted poor results in those cases with tibial intraarticular defects where the talus had a tendency to fall back into the residual tibial defect. This prompted the senior author to develop an intraarticular osteotomy known as the "plafondplasty" in an attempt to manage this challenging patient cohort.[25–27] The specific aim of plafondplasty is to realign the ankle joint by redistributing joint load from the affected medial/lateral side to the central and unaffected lateral/medial weight bearing surface of the tibial plafond. The defining feature of this osteotomy is that it is not above the deformity, as in the supramalleolar osteotomy, nor below the deformity, as in a calcaneal osteotomy or subtalar arthrodesis, but instead it is intraarticular. It is at the level of the deformity and so at the center of rotation and angulation. This avoids the creation of a secondary translational deformity, which is likely with supramalleolar and inframalleolar procedures when the correction is made intentionally at a level other than the center of rotation and angulation .

The plafondplasty is rarely indicated as an isolated procedure.[17,26,27] It is generally done with other soft tissue procedures to balance the joint. Occasionally, additional boney procedures—such as supramalleolar or inframalleolar osteotomies—are required. Reports on the use of a double osteotomy–supramalleolar with plafondplasty for asymmetric varus ankle OA seem to be promising.[28] The philosophy behind their use is that the plafondplasty rotates the medial impacted plafond along with restoring the alignment of the medial malleolus and the opening edge distal tibial supramalleolar osteotomy further shifts the mechanical axis laterally. There are now also reports on the use of a novel variant of the plafondplasty known as the "mortiseplasty," where an oblique medial distal tibial osteotomy without fibula osteotomy is performed.[29] The tibial osteotomy exits laterally in the plafond, that is, just extraarticularly. It is similarly able to correct the flattened orientation of the medial malleolus, and is particularly suited to asymmetric varus ankle OA with mortise widening because it results in a functional narrowing of the mortise (**Fig. 1**).

This article describes the authors' algorithm for the treatment of patients with asymmetric intraarticular varus and valgus ankle OA with the plafondplasty.

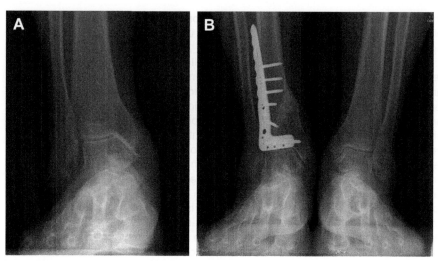

Fig. 1. (*A*) Varus ankle osteoarthritis demonstrating medial intraarticular erosion of the tibial plafond and flattening of the medial malleolus. (*B*) Correction achieved 1 year after mortiseplasty. (*Courtesy of* Professor Woo Chun Lee MD, Seoul, South Korea.)

PATIENT ASSESSMENT

Meticulous preoperative assessment is crucial. This starts with a detailed history taking particular note of prior trauma, symptoms of instability, previous surgery and complications thereof such as infection, and concomitant disease particularly diabetes and inflammatory arthropathy. Physical assessment commences with clinical gait analysis followed by examination of the patient in the standing position. This allows for evaluation of associated pelvic obliquity, limb length discrepancy, limb alignment, and heel varus or valgus. The skin should be assessed for scars and the viability of the soft tissue envelope. Palpation of the ankle, hind, mid, and forefoot is important to identify the location of any additional painful arthritic joints. Both active and passive range of motion of the ankle and subtalar joints should be assessed and documented. It is essential to remain vigilant for an associated Achilles tendon or gastrocnemius contracture, which may need to be addressed at the time of surgery. Ankle stability is tested with the patient seated, using standard talar tilt stress tests (inversion stress test for lateral and eversion stress test for medial ankle instability), and anterior drawer tests. The function of all tendons crossing the ankle joint should be tested. The posterior tibial tendon function is assessed with a single heel-rise test by observing hindfoot inversion. We recommend fluoroscopic assessment both in the office and then repeated intraoperatively. In varus deformity after reduction of the talus with passive manipulation and valgus stress, an indentation or intraarticular defect is seen over the medial aspect of the tibial articular surface (TAS). In valgus deformity, after reduction of the talus with passive manipulation and varus stress, the intraarticular defect is seen over the lateral aspect of the TAS. This groove or articular indentation results from increased and chronic contact pressure from the tilted talus within the plafond. These fluoroscopic stress tests are useful in all cases of asymmetric ankle OA because the distal tibial erosion often becomes much more evident on these views and can otherwise be overlooked (**Fig. 2**). It is imperative that the deformity is flexible and passively correctible, because the procedure is not indicated in fixed deformity.

We routinely use 4 weight-bearing radiographs including anteroposterior and lateral ankle, Mortise view, and a hindfoot alignment view. The mechanical axis and articular

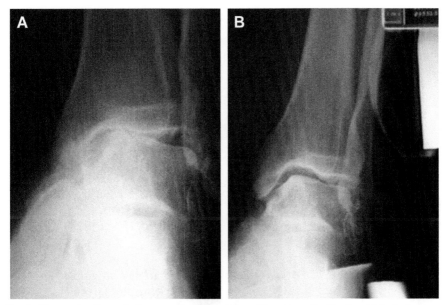

Fig. 2. The evaluation of all cases of asymmetric ankle osteoarthritis should include stress images. These help to both unmask any intraarticular deformity and also to confirm that the deformity is passively correctible. (*A*) (Weightbearing AP) demonstrates a typical intraarticular varus deformity. (*B*) (Stress View) demonstrates more clearly the erosion of the distal medial tibial plafond and that the ankle remains reducible. (*From* Myerson MS, Zide JR. Management of varus ankle osteoarthritis with joint-preserving osteotomy. Foot Ankle Clin 2013;18:474; with permission.)

angles are measured[18] (see **Fig. 2**). In patients with associated deformity elsewhere in the lower limb, full-leg length views should be obtained. To date, we do not routinely obtain preoperative computed tomography (CT), single photon-emission (SPECT)-CT/ CT, MRI, or diagnostic arthroscopy, although we recognize that these imaging modalities are advocated by some authors.[30–32] From a clinical perspective, we felt previously that these imaging modalities added little, because it is clear from plain radiographs that there is severe erosion. However, we now accept that there is a role for CT. From a clinical perspective, they facilitate more accurate preoperative planning of the osteotomy to the apex of the deformity than is possible with plain radiographs as these are frequently multiplanar deformities. Additionally, and from a research perspective, it would be interesting to know if any remodeling takes place within the intraarticular defects postoperatively. This detail would be best appreciated with CT scanning and to date there is no literature on this.

Traditional radiographic methods for assessing the mechanical alignment of the lower limb are unfortunately rarely useful in the planning of surgery for asymmetric ankle OA. This is because the traditional full limb length studies set the line from the center of the femoral head to the center of the tibial plafond.[33] Similarly, traditional hindfoot alignment radiographs only take into account nothing more proximal than the tibia.[34,35] The shortcomings of both of these methods are clear. What is really required for accurate preoperative planning in these cases is analysis of where the mechanical axis runs from the center of the femoral head to the lowest point of the calcaneus. A technique to describe this has recently been described, where full-length weight-bearing posteroanterior hip to calcaneus radiographs are obtained (**Fig. 3**).[36]

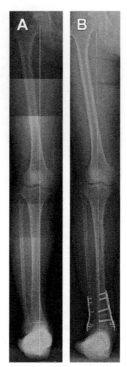

Fig. 3. Measurement of the weight bearing line in a hip to calcaneus radiograph.[36] (*A*) Preoperative. (*B*) Postoperative. (*Courtesy of* Naoki Haraguchi MD, Tokyo, Japan.)

This technique has been shown to have both high intraobserver and interobserver reliability and the preoperative values seem to be predictive of postoperative outcome. Of note, the authors also found concerns with the more traditionally use of the articular TAS angle (**Fig. 4**) for planning because, despite correcting the TAS angle correctly, consistently, and within an impressively narrow window, the postoperative weight-bearing point varied widely casting doubt on the usefulness of the TAS angle.[36]

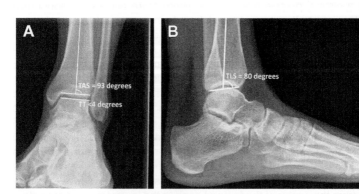

Fig. 4. Measurement of the (*A*) tibial ankle surface (TAS) angle (normal, 93°), talar tilt (TT) angle (normal, <4°) on an anteroposterior radiograph and (*B*) the tibial lateral surface (TLS) angle (normal, 80°).

OPERATIVE TECHNIQUE

We perform this operation as a day case procedure under general anesthesia and popliteal block for postoperative pain control. It is important to emphasize that the plafondplasty is rarely indicated in isolation and should be performed in conjunction with any required supramalleolar or inframalleolar realignment and stabilization. The etiology of the varus deformity is generally chronic lateral ankle instability. This leads to changes in the lateral stabilizers, and hence torn weak ligaments. Secondary changes occur in the peroneal tendons and the deformity progresses because of medial over pull. Because of this, a calcaneal osteotomy may also be necessary in addition to the lateral ligament stabilization procedure. On occasion, other medial bases procedures are necessary to balance the joint, as is the case in varus ankle arthroplasty, such as fractional posterior tibial tendon lengthening. Many surgeons would add an arthroscopic evaluation of the ankle joint to the procedure. However, the benefits of this are not obvious because diagnostically it is clear from plain radiographs that the joint is eroded and therapeutically the joint has minimal articular cartilage and these changes are too advanced for microfracture.

The patient is positioned supine and "bumped" appropriately, depending on whether a medial or lateral surgical approach is indicated. Fluoroscopic examination of the ankle is repeated to ensure that the deformity is flexible with appropriate varus or valgus stress centering the talus. In addition any associated medial and or lateral instability are reevaluated more accurately in this setting than in the office. Lateral instability is almost invariably present in asymmetric intraarticular varus ankle OA and it is important to maintain a high index of suspicion for concomitant medial instability in these cases too. Although counterintuitive, the chronic medial abutment associated with these varus cases can lead to severe deltoid ligament attenuation. Conversely, on occasion, the deltoid ligament can require release in long-standing varus cases. In our experience to date, medial insufficiency is rarely encountered in asymmetric intraarticular valgus OA.

The position of the incisions should take into account the planned osteotomy and any additional procedures required. Regardless of whether it is a varus or valgus deformity, always start laterally. Evaluate the peroneal tendons and lateral ankle joint, and remove any lateral gutter osteophytes that will block reduction of the joint.

In varus and valgus cases, extraperiosteal dissection is performed. The apex of the osteotomy is directed toward the intraarticular deformity from the medial or lateral aspect of the distal tibia. A Kirschner wire is initially used as a guide to the plane of the osteotomy and aimed at the apex of the intraarticular deformity (**Fig. 5**). We have previously templated preoperatively based on plain radiographs but, as stated, we are increasingly relying on preoperative CT scanning to determine more accurately the apex of the deformity, which is so rarely in a single plane. It cannot be emphasized enough that the placement of the osteotomy guide wire is critical and every effort should be made to center it perfectly at the apex. If there is any doubt, it is best to err on the side of placing the wire just beyond the apex or to cut on the far side of the wire because it is essential to not underestimate the location of the apex. Two or 3 additional Kirschner wires are then introduced parallel to the joint surface of the tibial plafond within the subchondral bone just under the articular cartilage at the apex of the plafond angulation. These act to prevent penetration of the saw blade into the joint during the osteotomy and as a hinge during the deformity correction (**Fig. 6**). The osteotomy is performed with an oscillating saw, which is perpendicular to the anteroposterior axis of the tibia and in the same plane as the guide Kirschner wire. It ends at the level of the previously inserted blocking Kirschner wires,

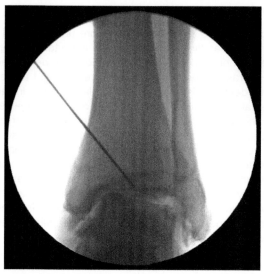

Fig. 5. A Kirschner wire is used initially as a guide to the plane of the osteotomy and aimed at the apex of the intraarticular deformity.

thus keeping the subchondral bone bridge intact. The orientation of the saw blade is critical during the osteotomy. Because the cut is made along the length of the guide wire, it is essential to check the rotation of the blade to ensure that it is not cutting more either anteriorly or posteriorly. If the cut is performed with malrotation, it will not end precisely at the apex of the deformity and the osteotomy will be compromised. The bone bridge and the blocking Kirschner wires are then used as a hinge along with a broad osteotome to gradually lever open the plafond until the respective medial or lateral TAS is parallel to the intact portion of the distal tibia. At this point, a lamina spreader is inserted into the cortical gap (**Fig. 7**) to hold the correction while cancellous bone chips are inserted into the defect to maintain a parallel joint surface. In contrast with supramalleolar osteotomies where a slight overcorrection of the deformity is often desirable in plafondplasty a precise correction is required—with undercorrection or overcorrection being undesirable. For fixation, screws in isolation

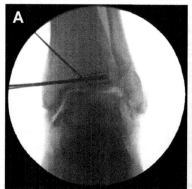
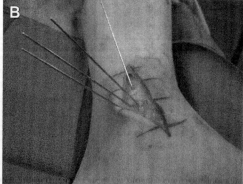

Fig. 6. (*A, B*) The parallel wires act to prevent penetration of the saw blade into the joint during the osteotomy and as a hinge during the deformity correction.

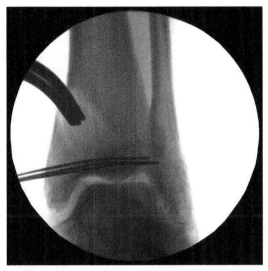

Fig. 7. A lamina spreader is inserted into the cortical gap to hold the correction while cancellous bone chips are inserted into the defect.

can be used but a plate is generally preferable. This does not need to be a locking plate and it is generally preferable to avoid using too rigid a construct. The plate serves both as a buttress and to keep the bone graft in place (**Fig. 8**). If the osteotomy breaches the articular surface or there is any (even minimal) displacement at the level of the plafond then it is necessary to insert 1 or 2 screws across the most distal subchondral of the joint to hold the position.

For intraarticular varus deformity, lateral ankle instability is invariably encountered. This instability is corrected with a modified Chrisman Snook procedure.[37] The decision to perform ligament reconstruction should be made before the plafondplasty is

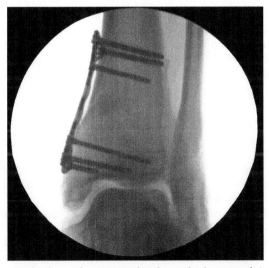

Fig. 8. The plate serves both as a buttress and to keep the bone graft in place.

performed and is based on the extent of instability present. The peroneus brevis tendon is split and passed through the fibula. However, it is not tensioned until the osteotomy for the plafondplasty is completed. As mentioned, it is essential to screen for and treat any associated concomitant medial instability. For intraarticular valgus deformity, insufficiency of the deltoid is theoretically possible, but is rarely encountered. These valgus deformities tend to reduce easily when the osteotomy is hinged open from the lateral side and medial ankle joint does not book open, as is commonly seen in stage IV flatfoot deformity.

During the procedure, it is imperative to ensure that any excess bone, osteophyte, or debris present in the gutters are resected adequately. This is particularly frequently required in cases with associated lateral ankle instability. For the lateral gutter, the debridement is performed through the lateral incision used for the modified Chrisman Snook procedure. To date, we have not found a formal medial gutter debridement to be required, even in the valgus cases.

Postoperatively, the limb is placed in a below-knee Jones type splint for the first 2 weeks, followed by the application of a removable boot with instructions to remain nonweightbearing, but to perform active range of motion exercises for 5 minutes 5 times daily. At 6 weeks patients, are encouraged to commence partial weight bearing of 50 pounds of body weight, and at 8 weeks, full weight bearing is permitted. The removable boot is worn for a total of 10 to 12 weeks, depending on the rate of healing of the osteotomy.

The senior author has previously reported promising medium term data for the plafondplasty in intraarticular varus ankles with significant improvements in varus tilt and American Orthopaedic Foot and Ankle Society scores at a mean of 59 months.[26]

SUMMARY

Asymmetric ankle OA is an increasingly recognized condition. It is imperative to differentiate between extraarticular and intraarticular deformity and to address these appropriately. Additionally, any associated instability and multilevel deformity must be recognized and addressed. Patients with intraarticular varus or valgus asymmetric OA have poorer outcomes and higher rates of recurrence when treated with standard techniques targeted at correction with traditional supramalleolar or inframalleolar techniques. In contrast, plafondplasty aims to correct the deformity at its center of rotation and angulation and is associated with low rates of recurrence, substantial postoperative pain relief, functional improvement, and a possible slowing of the degenerative process.

REFERENCES

1. Cushnaghan J, Dieppe P. Study of 500 patients with limb joint osteoarthritis. I. Analysis by age, sex, and distribution of symptomatic joint sites. Ann Rheum Dis 1991;50:8–13.
2. Goldberg AJ, MacGregor A, Dawson J, et al. The demand incidence of symptomatic ankle osteoarthritis presenting to foot & ankle surgeons in the United Kingdom. Foot (Edinb) 2012;22:163–6.
3. Woolf AD, Pfleger B. Burden of major musculoskeletal conditions. Bull World Health Organ 2003;81:646–56.
4. Woolf AD, Akesson K. Understanding the burden of musculoskeletal conditions. The burden is huge and not reflected in national health priorities. BMJ 2001;322:1079–80.

5. Glazebrook M, Daniels T, Younger A, et al. Comparison of health-related quality of life between patients with end-stage ankle and hip arthrosis. J Bone Joint Surg Am 2008;90:499–505.
6. Saltzman CL, Salamon ML, Blanchard GM, et al. Epidemiology of ankle arthritis: report of a consecutive series of 639 patients from a tertiary orthopaedic center. Iowa Orthop J 2005;25:44–6.
7. Valderrabano V, Horisberger M, Russell I, et al. Etiology of ankle osteoarthritis. Clin Orthop Relat Res 2009;467:1800–6.
8. Golditz T, Steib S, Pfeifer K, et al. Functional ankle instability as a risk factor for osteoarthritis: using T2-mapping to analyze early cartilage degeneration in the ankle joint of young athletes. Osteoarthr Cartil 2014;22:1377–85.
9. Harrington KD. Degenerative arthritis of the ankle secondary to long-standing lateral ligament instability. J Bone Joint Surg Am 1979;61:354–61.
10. Horisberger M, Valderrabano V, Hintermann B. Posttraumatic ankle osteoarthritis after ankle-related fractures. J Orthop Trauma 2009;23:60–7.
11. Knupp M, Stufkens SA, van Bergen CJ, et al. Effect of supramalleolar varus and valgus deformities on the tibiotalar joint: a cadaveric study. Foot Ankle Int 2011; 32:609–15.
12. Pagenstert GI, Hintermann B, Barg A, et al. Realignment surgery as alternative treatment of varus and valgus ankle osteoarthritis. Clin Orthop Relat Res 2007; 462:156–68.
13. Pagenstert G, Knupp M, Valderrabano V, et al. Realignment surgery for valgus ankle osteoarthritis. Oper Orthop Traumatol 2009;21:77–87.
14. Wang B, Saltzman CL, Chalayon O, et al. Does the subtalar joint compensate for ankle malalignment in end-stage ankle arthritis? Clin Orthop Relat Res 2015;473: 318–25.
15. Kura H, Kitaoka HB, Luo ZP, et al. Measurement of surface contact area of the ankle joint. Clin Biomech (Bristol, Avon) 1998;13:365–70.
16. Lee KB, Cho YJ. Oblique supramalleolar opening wedge osteotomy without fibular osteotomy for varus deformity of the ankle. Foot Ankle Int 2009;30:565–7.
17. Stamatis ED, Cooper PS, Myerson MS. Supramalleolar osteotomy for the treatment of distal tibial angular deformities and arthritis of the ankle joint. Foot Ankle Int 2003;24:754–64.
18. Benthien RA, Myerson MS. Supramalleolar osteotomy for ankle deformity and arthritis. Foot Ankle Clin 2004;9:475–87, viii.
19. Takakura Y, Takaoka T, Tanaka Y, et al. Results of opening-wedge osteotomy for the treatment of a post-traumatic varus deformity of the ankle. J Bone Joint Surg Am 1998;80:213–8.
20. Tanaka Y, Takakura Y, Hayashi K, et al. Low tibial osteotomy for varus-type osteoarthritis of the ankle. J Bone Joint Surg Br 2006;88:909–13.
21. Abraham E, Lubicky JP, Songer MN, et al. Supramalleolar osteotomy for ankle valgus in myelomeningocele. J Pediatr Orthop 1996;16:774–81.
22. Coester LM, Saltzman CL, Leupold J, et al. Long-term results following ankle arthrodesis for post-traumatic arthritis. J Bone Joint Surg Am 2001;83-A:219–28.
23. Kumar SJ, Keret D, MacEwen GD. Corrective cosmetic supramalleolar osteotomy for valgus deformity of the ankle joint: a report of two cases. J Pediatr Orthop 1990;10:124–7.
24. Malhotra D, Puri R, Owen R. Valgus deformity of the ankle in children with spina bifida aperta. J Bone Joint Surg Br 1984;66:381–5.
25. Becker AS, Myerson MS. The indications and technique of supramalleolar osteotomy. Foot Ankle Clin 2009;14:549–61.

26. Mann HA, Filippi J, Myerson MS. Intra-articular opening medial tibial wedge osteotomy (plafond-plasty) for the treatment of intra-articular varus ankle arthritis and instability. Foot Ankle Int 2012;33:255–61.
27. Myerson MS, Zide JR. Management of varus ankle osteoarthritis with joint-preserving osteotomy. Foot Ankle Clin 2013;18:471–80.
28. Hintermann BKM, Barg A. Novel double osteotomy of distal tibia for correction of asymmetric varus osteoarthritic ankle. Chicago: American Academy of Orthopedic Surgeons; 2013. Available at: www.aaos.org.
29. Ahn T, Yi Y, Cho J, et al. A cohort study of patients undergoing distal tibial osteotomy without fibula osteotomy for medial ankle arthritis with mortise widening. J Bone Joint Surg Am 2015;97(5):381–8.
30. Valderrabano V, Paul J, Horisberger M, et al. Joint-preserving surgery of valgus ankle osteoarthritis. Foot Ankle Clin 2013;18:481–502.
31. Pagenstert GI, Barg A, Leumann AG, et al. SPECT-CT imaging in degenerative joint disease of the foot and ankle. J Bone Joint Surg Br 2009;91:1191–6.
32. Chhabra A, Soldatos T, Chalian M, et al. Current concepts review: 3T magnetic resonance imaging of the ankle and foot. Foot Ankle Int 2012;33:164–71.
33. Paley D. Principles of deformity correction. New York: Springer-Verlag; 2002. p. 19–30.
34. Cobey JC. Posterior roentgenogram of the foot. Clin Orthop Relat Res 1976;(118):202–7.
35. Saltzman CL, el-Khoury GY. The hindfoot alignment view. Foot Ankle Int 1995;16:572–6.
36. Haraguchi N, Ota K, Tsunoda N, et al. Weight-bearing-line analysis in supramalleolar osteotomy for varus-type osteoarthritis of the ankle. J Bone Joint Surg Am 2015;97:333–9.
37. Acevedo JI, Myerson MS. Modification of the Chrisman-Snook technique. Foot Ankle Int 2000;21:154–5.

Extraarticular Supramalleolar Osteotomy for Managing Varus Ankle Osteoarthritis, Alternatives for Osteotomy: How and Why?

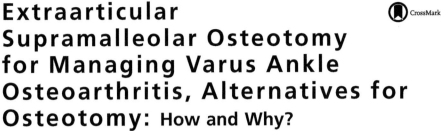

Woo-Chun Lee, MD, PhD

KEYWORDS

• Osteoarthritis • Supramalleolar osteotomy • Varus ankle osteoarthritis

KEY POINTS

- A conventional supramalleolar osteotomy cannot restore parallel joint lines between the tibial plafond and talar dome in ankles with a large talar tilt.
- The distal tibial oblique osteotomy was introduced because a more horizontal supramalleolar osteotomy cannot stabilize a joint with mortise widening.
- Talar tilt does not change after distal tibial oblique osteotomy; however, medial and lateral gutters become congruent by narrowing of the ankle mortise after osteotomy.
- Knowledge of the 3-dimensional structural change in the ankle mortise and the talus may be critical for further improvement of joint-preserving surgery.

INTRODUCTION

An opening or closing wedge supramalleolar osteotomy may be indicated to address traumatic malunion, or congenital or residual coronal plane deformity.[1–5] Previous articles have reported the supramalleolar osteotomy as a joint preserving surgery with good clinical outcome for asymmetric ankle osteoarthritis, especially varus ankle osteoarthritis.[1–6] However, clinical and radiologic outcome have been reported as unsatisfactory in varus ankle osteoarthritis with large talar tilt or obliteration of joint space between the tibial plafond and talar dome.[1,5] Patients with partial joint space narrowing or obliteration may not show a good result after conventional, more horizontal

The author has nothing to disclose.
Department of Orthopaedic Surgery, Seoul Foot and Ankle Center, Seoul Paik Hospital, Inje University, 85, 2-ga, Jeo-dong, Jung-gu, Seoul 100-032, South Korea
E-mail address: leewoochun@gmail.com

supramalleolar osteotomies. An ankle with medial gutter narrowing with no or minimal talar tilt generally shows good results. However, an ankle with large talar tilt or widening of the ankle mortise often fails after supramalleolar osteotomy (**Fig. 1**).

Supramalleolar osteotomy of the tibia and fibula creates angulation and translation of the ankle joint without changing the width of the ankle mortise. Therefore, when there is ankle osteoarthritis with mortise widening, supramalleolar osteotomy cannot achieve a stable bony mortise. To achieve a stable mortise after osteotomy in an ankle with mortise widening, only the distal tibia needs to be angulated without osteotomy of the fibula.

The ankle joint has a stable structure in which translation of the talus is blocked by the medial and lateral malleoli. However, under circumstances such as syndesmosis diastasis, fibular fracture, or malalignment resulting in mortise widening, the talus loses its stability and moves laterally within the ankle joint. Biomechanical studies have shown that the lateral translation of the talus results in reducing tibiotalar contact area[7] thus creating a nonphysiologic load distribution within the ankle joint.

The mortise widening that affects stability of the ankle joint can also occur in some cases of medial ankle osteoarthritis. As medial ankle osteoarthritis progresses, the talus migrates to the medial side of the ankle joint causing medial joint space narrowing, which may result eventually in erosion of the medial malleolus and mortise widening (**Fig. 2**). Through widening the ankle, the mortise and talus become incongruent and narrowing of the ankle mortise is necessary to restore congruity. Ankle mortise widening is the result of intraarticular erosion in most cases as shown in **Fig. 2**. However, in ankles without contact of bony surfaces in the medial gutter such as stage 2 of the Takakura classification, it may suggest some developmental widening. To treat

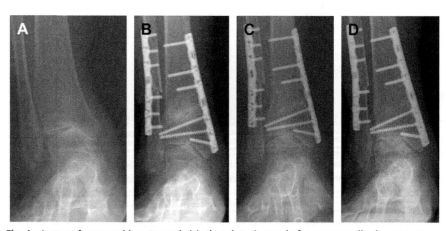

Fig. 1. A case of varus ankle osteoarthritis that deteriorated after supramalleolar osteotomy. (*A*) The preoperative anteroposterior radiograph shows marked widening of the ankle mortise and obliteration of the medial gutter. The tibial plafond–talar dome joint space was preserved and talar tilt angle was 9.5°. (*B*) Two months postoperatively, the anteroposterior radiograph shows valgus angulation of the tibial plafond, widening of the medial gutter and contact between medial aspect of the tibial plafond and talar dome. (*C*) One year postoperatively, the radiograph shows progression of degenerative changes with sclerosis and cystic changes at the contact point of the tibial plafond and the talus. The talar tilt was 18.5°. (*D*) Radiographs taken 2.5 years postoperatively showing deterioration of osteoarthritis with almost complete obliteration of the tibial plafond–talar dome joint space. The talar tilt decreased to 11.5°.

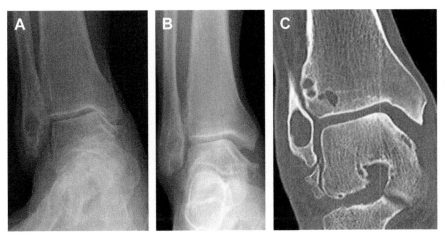

Fig. 2. A case of varus ankle osteoarthritis with erosion of the medial malleolus. (*A*) The anteroposterior weight-bearing radiograph shows medial translation of the talus relative to the tibia and medial gutter obliteration. (*B*) A non–weight-bearing anteroposterior radiograph shows widening of the medial gutter and suspicious erosion of the medial malleolus. (*C*) A coronal computed tomography image shows complete erosion of the articular facet of the medial malleolus about 2 mm inferior to the tibial plafond.

medial ankle osteoarthritis with mortise widening, restoration of width and shape of ankle mortise as well as lateral shifting of weight-bearing axis are required.

Plafondplasty has been suggested as a method to correct the alignment of the tibial plafond and it also can narrow the width of ankle mortise,[8] because it angulates only the medial part of the tibial plafond. However, plafondplasty is an intraarticular osteotomy that is indicated when there is deformity in the tibial plafond. Therefore, another method of distal tibial osteotomy was developed.[9] In this procedure, the osteotomized distal fragment is shifted inferolaterally using the lateral apex of the osteotomy as a hinge (**Fig. 3**).

PREOPERATIVE PLANNING FOR DISTAL TIBIAL OBLIQUE OSTEOTOMY
Assessment of Mortise Widening

Ankle mortise widening is determined by weight-bearing radiographs and confirmed intraoperatively. Mortise widening is suspected if the medial clear space on valgus stress radiographs is greater than 3 mm.[9,10] Mortise widening is measured as the shortest distance between the medial surface of the talus at the level of the talar dome and the lateral surface of the medial malleolus.[9] Some individuals may have widened medial clear space on a valgus stress view after deltoid ligament injury. However, widening of medial clear space in deltoid injury is usually accompanied by valgus talar tilt, which is different from medial clear space widening without or with minimal talar tilt in ankles with mortise widening. When mortise widening is suspected without large widening of medial clear space on a valgus stress view, widening of the medial clear space is assessed again intraoperatively, with valgus stress under anesthesia after exposure of the medial gutter.

Assessment of the Medial Translation of the Talus

A concept of the center of the talus was developed to evaluate the translation of the talus within the ankle mortise preoperatively and postoperatively.[9] The center of the

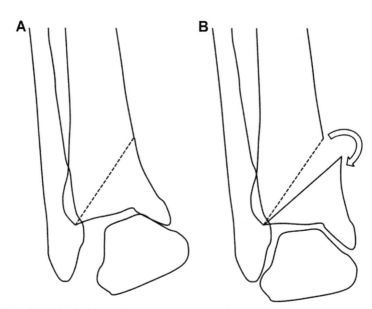

Fig. 3. The distal tibial oblique osteotomy. (*A*) An oblique osteotomy is planned along the line connecting a point at the medial tibial cortex 5 cm proximal to the ankle joint and a point at the lateral tibial cortex at 5 mm above the joint. (*B*) The ankle mortise becomes narrow as the distal fragment is displaced inferiorly. Geometrically, talar tilt increases because tibial plafond is more angulated relative to the talar dome.

talus is defined as being located along a line connecting the medial and lateral malleolus. It is also assumed that a circle originating from the center of the talus is tangential to the midpoint of the talar dome (**Fig. 4**). The talus center migration is measured on a weight-bearing anteroposterior view. Talus center migration was defined as the shortest distance between the tibial axis to the center of talus. When the talus center translated 3 mm or more, it is considered as evidence of ankle mortise widening.

SURGICAL TECHNIQUE OF DISTAL TIBIAL OBLIQUE OSTEOTOMY

In earlier cases, the osteotomy was performed through a medial approach. However, an anterior midline approach has been used in later cases owing to difficulties with applying a plate on medial cortex after opening the osteotomy site. Another reason for changing the approach was the difficulty of osteotomizing the lateral aspect of the tibia. In contrast with the conventional supramalleolar osteotomy, the distal tibial oblique osteotomy should continue through the lateral cortex to prevent fracture into the joint while opening the osteotomy site.

A longitudinal incision is made along the anterior midline of the ankle 10 cm proximal to 5 cm distal to the joint (**Fig. 5**). Further dissection is done between the extensor hallucis longus and extensor digitorum longus for exposure of the distal tibia. An oblique osteotomy is performed as planned along the line connecting a point at medial tibial cortex 5 cm proximal to the ankle joint and a point at lateral tibial cortex at 5 mm above the joint. After insertion of 2 or 3 Kirschner wires along the planned osteotomy line, the position of the Kirschner wires is confirmed by fluoroscopy. Multiple holes are made along the planned osteotomy line, and then the osteotomy is completed connecting the holes using a thin osteotome. After spreading the osteotomy using the lateral

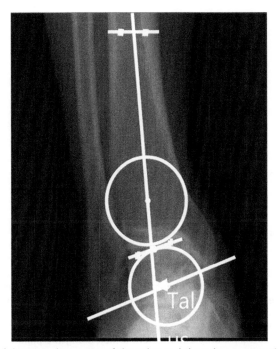

Fig. 4. Method of drawing the center of the talus and the talus–center migration. The center of the talus was defined as being located along a line connecting the medial and lateral malleolus. It was also assumed that a circle originating from the center of the talus is tangential to the midpoint of the talar dome. Talus–center migration was defined as the shortest distance between the tibial axis to the center of talus.

apex as a hinge to shift the distal tibial fragment inferiorly, a locking plate is applied for stabilization. Autogenous iliac bone graft, both cancellous and cortical, is packed into the defect. Postoperatively, a non–weight-bearing short leg cast is applied for 6 weeks After that, weight bearing is allowed in a short leg splint or ankle–foot orthosis, depending on the consolidation of the osteotomy.

Complications

In the author's practice, hardware removal was necessary more frequently in patients in whom the medial approach was used. An intraarticular osteotomy was made inadvertently in one of the ankles approached from medial. The distal tibiofibular syndesmosis was widened and the distal tibial fragment was transfixed to the fibula intraoperatively in a few ankles.

Patients with mortise widening of less than 4 mm often experience lateral bony impingement postoperatively. Therefore, lateral impingement should be expected when applied to patients with mortise widening less than 4 mm and preemptive lateral spur excision may be required.

Necessity of Lateral Ligament Reconstruction

Lateral ligament reconstruction has been regarded by some authors as an important step of treatment for medial ankle osteoarthritis because lateral instability is known as a common cause of medial ankle osteoarthritis.[8,11–13] In contrast, other authors felt

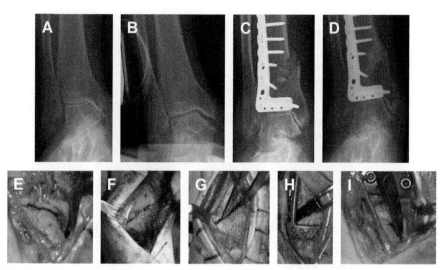

Fig. 5. Surgical technique of the distal tibial oblique osteotomy. (*A*) Preoperative weight-bearing radiograph showing medial gutter obliteration. (*B*) Preoperative valgus stress view showing widening of medial gutter. (*C*) Immediate postoperative and (*D*) 1 year postoperative radiographs showing restoration of the medial clear space and a congruent lateral gutter. (*E*) Intraoperative photograph showing widening of the medial gutter on abduction of the foot. (*F*) Multiple holes were drilled along the planned osteotomy line. (*G*) Osteotomy was completed with small osteotomes. (*H*) A locking plate was applied after opening of the osteotomy. (*I*) There is no gap in the medial gutter on abduction of the foot after opening at the osteotomy site.

that treatment of chronic lateral ankle instability is not important in the result of realignment surgery and chronic instability disappears after shifting of weight-bearing load to the lateral aspect of the ankle.[3,5] Osteoarthritis may have developed as a result of chronic ankle instability in some ankles of the author's series of more than 100 distal tibial osteotomies, which can be concluded from the history of chronic instability and a talar tilt of more than 10° in the preoperative varus stress test. However, if the lateral gutter is congruent on postoperative weight-bearing anteroposterior radiographs, then lateral ligament reconstruction would not further decrease the talar tilt. Even if talar tilt persisted after surgery, no patient complained of lateral ankle instability postoperatively; thus, the talar tilt on the postoperative radiograph may be considered as a result of an increased slant of the tibial plafond owing to distal tibial oblique osteotomy. In essence, we do not think that lateral ligament reconstruction is essential for successful results after Mortiseplasty. On the other hand, hindfoot varus may also cause medial ankle osteoarthritis. However, heel varus was not so large in the author's series, in which mean preoperative hindfoot varus was 5.2° and changed to 2.1° postoperatively.[9] Lateral impingement rather than residual hindfoot varus may be a problem after distal tibial osteotomy[1]; therefore, an additional calcaneal osteotomy to correct the hindfoot varus was not considered.

RESULTS OF DISTAL TIBIAL OBLIQUE OSTEOTOMY

Mean talar tilt did not decrease significantly after distal tibial oblique osteotomy, whereas clinical scores and radiographic stage improved in most patients.[9] Talar tilt increased in 6 of 18 ankles, and among them it increased by more than 2° in 4 ankles.

The absolute value of preoperative talar tilt that will still be associated for a good prognosis could not be determined from this study. Distal tibial oblique osteotomy narrows the ankle mortise while slanting the tibial plafond relative to the talar dome. In contrast with the conventional supramalleolar osteotomy of the tibia and fibula, talar tilt can be increased after distal tibial oblique osteotomy. Thus, the preoperative talar tilt adequate for distal tibial oblique osteotomy may be smaller than the previously suggested limit for supramalleolar osteotomy, which was either 7.3° or 10°. However, distal tibial oblique osteotomy may be used as an interim procedure to delay definitive surgery for ankles with substantial talar tilt, because excellent clinical results were obtained in ankles with more than 7° of talar tilt in the current study and there is a report of good clinical results in ankles with a mean talar tilt of about 10°.[11]

Mean talar tilt in this series was 5.6° preoperatively and 5.5° postoperatively. We, therefore, concluded that ankles with minimal talar tilt are indicated for this surgery.

Difference of Ankle Geometry After Distal Tibial Oblique Osteotomy Compared with Supramalleolar Osteotomy

In distal tibial oblique osteotomy, the amount of shifting of the osteotomized fragment is limited by the fibula, whereas supramalleolar osteotomy achieves a greater amount of shifting of the weight-bearing axis through an additional fibular osteotomy. However, adequate correction of tibial plafond was achieved in our patients and talus center migration also proved that the center of the talus moved laterally after distal tibial oblique osteotomy. In supramalleolar osteotomy of the tibia and fibula the shape of the ankle mortise remains unchanged; however, in distal tibial oblique osteotomy, the shape of the ankle mortise is changed and the tibial plafond is slanted more relative to the talar dome.

With supramalleolar osteotomy, a widened lateral gutter is not becoming congruent. In distal tibial oblique osteotomy, the preoperative widening of the lateral gutter disappears with restoration of congruency between the articular surfaces of the lateral malleolus and the talus. Increased slating of the tibial plafond is responsible for the residual talar tilt after distal tibial oblique osteotomy. If the talar tilt after distal tibial oblique osteotomy is caused by lateral instability, the lateral gutter should be widened inferiorly.

SUMMARY

The supramalleolar osteotomy has been reported to be a joint preserving surgery with good clinical outcome for asymmetric ankle osteoarthritis, especially varus ankle osteoarthritis. However, in case of varus ankle osteoarthritis with large talar tilt or obliteration of joint space between the tibial plafond and talar dome, clinical and radiologic outcome have been reported as not satisfactory.[1,5]

Conventional supramalleolar osteotomy of the tibia and fibula creates angulation and translation of the ankle joint without changing the width of the ankle mortise. Therefore, when there is ankle osteoarthritis with mortise widening, supramalleolar osteotomy cannot reestablish a stable bony mortise (see **Fig. 1**). For this the distal tibia needs to be angulated without fibular osteotomy.

Plafondplasty can correct the alignment of the tibial plafond and it also narrows the ankle mortise,[8] however it bears the risk of an intraarticular osteotomy and maybe indicated for a deformity in the tibial plafond. Therefore another method of distal tibial osteotomy was developed.[9] In this procedure, the osteotomized distal fragment is shifted inferolaterally using the lateral apex of the osteotomy as a hinge.

Distal tibial oblique osteotomy improved the preoperative clinical and radiological parameters; however, mean talar tilt angle did not decrease. Therefore it may be indicated in an ankle osteoarthritis with mortise widening with small degree of talar tilt (up to 7°).[1]

Conventional joint-sparing surgery for the ankle was not successful in restoration of parallel alignment of the tibial plafond and talar dome. The rationale behind the current method of joint-sparing surgery is to restore ankle stability by shifting of the weight-bearing load to the other side of the ankle with intact articular cartilage, or to restore the stability of the ankle by contouring of the ankle mortise to fit the shape of the talus. This rationale has been developed from an idea to normalize an ankle geometry based on the coronal plane assessment.

Only 1 article reported restoration of parallel joint lines in ankles with large degree of talar tilt.[14] The patients in that series had a long standing paralytic cavovarus deformity. Mean preoperative talar tilt was 17.4°, and it decreased to 1.4° at a mean follow-up of 3 years. In that series, restoration of the plantigrade foot and dynamic balancing by tendon transfer was the reason of the success of joint sparing surgery in ankles with a large talar tilt. Tendon transfers resulted in weakening of the invertors and strengthening of evertors, which means 3-dimensional correction of the foot and ankle. Therefore, assessment of ankle arthritis in sagittal, axial, and coronal planes may be helpful to achieve a decrease of the talar tilt in ankle osteoarthritis.

REFERENCES

1. Lee WC, Moon JS, Lee K, et al. Indications for supramalleolar osteotomy in patients with ankle osteoarthritis and varus deformity. J Bone Joint Surg Am 2011; 93(13):1243–8.
2. Pagenstert GI, Hintermann B, Barg A, et al. Realignment surgery as alternative treatment of varus and valgus ankle osteoarthritis. Clin Orthop Relat Res 2007; 462:156–68.
3. Takakura Y, Tanaka Y, Kumai T, et al. Low tibial osteotomy for osteoarthritis of the ankle. Results of a new operation in 18 patients. J Bone Joint Surg Br 1995;77(1): 50–4.
4. Takakura Y, Takaoka T, Tanaka Y, et al. Results of opening-wedge osteotomy for the treatment of a post-traumatic varus deformity of the ankle. J Bone Joint Surg Am 1998;80(2):213–8.
5. Tanaka Y, Takakura Y, Hayashi K, et al. Low tibial osteotomy for varus-type osteoarthritis of the ankle. J Bone Joint Surg Br 2006;88(7):909–13.
6. Stamatis ED, Cooper PS, Myerson MS. Supramalleolar osteotomy for the treatment of distal tibial angular deformities and arthritis of the ankle joint. Foot Ankle Int 2003;24(10):754–64.
7. Ramsey PL, Hamilton W. Changes in tibiotalar area of contact caused by lateral talar shift. J Bone Joint Surg Am 1976;58(3):356–7.
8. Mann HA, Filippi J, Myerson MS. Intra-articular opening medial tibial wedge osteotomy (plafond-plasty) for the treatment of intra-articular varus ankle arthritis and instability. Foot Ankle Int 2012;33(4):255–61.
9. Ahn TK, Yi Y, Cho JH, et al. A cohort study of patients undergoing distal tibial osteotomy without fibular osteotomy for medial ankle arthritis with mortise widening. J Bone Joint Surg Am 2015;97(5):381–8.
10. Park SS, Kubiak EN, Egol KA, et al. Stress radiographs after ankle fracture: The effect of ankle position and deltoid ligament status on medial clear space measurements. J Orthop Trauma 2006;20(1):11–8.

11. Lee HS, Wapner KL, Park SS, et al. Ligament reconstruction and calcaneal osteotomy for osteoarthritis of the ankle. Foot Ankle Int 2009;30(6):475–80.
12. Harrington KD. Degenerative arthritis of the ankle secondary to long-standing lateral ligament instability. J Bone Joint Surg Am 1979;61(3):354–61.
13. Valderrabano V, Hintermann B, Horisberger M, et al. Ligamentous posttraumatic ankle osteoarthritis. Am J Sports Med 2006;34(4):612–20.
14. Lee WC, Ahn JY, Cho JH, et al. Realignment surgery for severe talar tilt secondary to paralytic cavovarus. Foot Ankle Int 2013;34(11):1552–9.

Corrective Osteotomies for Malunited Malleolar Fractures

Daniel Weber, MD[a], Martin Weber, MD[b],*

KEYWORDS

- Ankle fracture • Ankle malunion • Osteotomy malleolus

KEY POINTS

- Malunions after malleolar fractures lead to joint instability and result in abnormal weight transfer that can cause arthritic joint destruction.
- The initial morphology of the instability cause by the fractures and the ligamentous lesions will also be found in the malunion.
- After documentation of the malunion a treatment plan has to be drawn up addressing soft tissues, osteotomies, osteosynthesis, implants, and rehabilitation.
- Correction includes the malunited medial and lateral malleolus as well as the posterior tibial rim.

INTRODUCTION: NATURE OF THE PROBLEM

The primary goal of ankle fracture treatment is reconstruction of a congruent joint surface and restoration of stability and anatomic alignment. Ankle fractures are very common and most of these injuries heal very well. However, some of these fractures fail to consolidate and become nonunions (see Capogna BM, Egol KA: Treatment of Nonunions After Malleolar Fractures, in this issue). Others heal in nonanatomic positions and are called malunions. Malunions can occur in diaphyseal and articular fractures. In diaphyseal malunions shortening, angulation, and/or malrotation can be present.

Irregularities of the joint surface are present in malunions of articular fractures. Both types of malunions result in abnormal weight transfer and can cause arthritic joint destruction. The instability in a fracture is defined by the loss of bony guidance, ruptured ligaments, and disturbed coaptation (**Figs. 1–4**). Even a minor lateral

The authors have nothing to disclose.
[a] Department of Orthopaedics and Traumatology, St. Claraspital, Kleinriehenstrasse 30, 4016 Basel, Switzerland; [b] Department of Orthopaedics and Traumatology, Siloah AG, Worbstrasse 316, 3073 Gümligen, Switzerland
* Corresponding author.
E-mail address: Martin.Weber@spitalnetzbern.ch

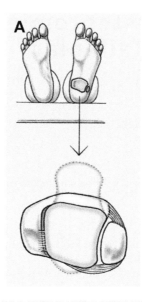

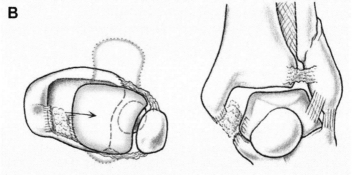

Fig. 1. (*A, B*): The left ankle. (*A*) View from below. (*B*) Anterior view. Rupture of the deltoid ligament, widened joint space, rupture of the anterior tibiofibular ligament, fracture of the lateral malleolus with shortening and external rotation, translation of the talus. (*From Weber D, Borisch N, Weber M. Treatment of malunion in ankle fractures. Eur J Trauma Emerg Surg 2010;36:522; with permission.*)

translation of the talus of 1 mm leads to a decrease of the articular contact surface of 42%[1] (**Fig. 5**). Translation and rotation of the talus increase this phenomenon.

Malunions are caused by misjudged fracture instability and therefore inadequate fixation, inappropriate surgical technique, inaccurate reduction, and/or secondary dislocation of fracture fragments. This applies to both surgical and nonsurgical fracture treatment.

Clinically, malunions lead to joint instability. This instability can be managed in minor deformities by strengthening of the extrinsic muscles and proprioceptive training. In cases with severe deformity, arthritic changes, poor muscular performance, and in high demand patients, symptoms such as pain, swelling, and functional impairment are present in various degrees. In these cases, correction of the malunion may be indicated. The patient's age, occupation, and range of motion have to be evaluated when

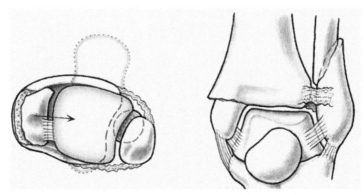

Fig. 2. Typical anatomy of a malunited bimalleolar fracture with lateral translation of the talus. Owing to the horizontal fracture line of the medial malleolus, the displacement may be difficult to see because the medial "clear space" and the angle of the malleolus to the plafond are not altered. The lateral malleolus is rotated externally and shortened and the lateral edge of the plafond may show impaction, usually posteriorly.

considering surgery. It is not the severity of arthritic changes as seen in radiographs that indicates the need for surgery. Pain is the most important indication for surgery.

OPERATIVE TECHNIQUE

It is important to understand the pathologic anatomy of the malunion. It is defined by the initial trauma and the lesions that have occurred, that is, the morphology of and instability caused by the fractures and ligamentous lesions will also be found in the malunion, both in the case of untreated fractures and fractures treated with inadequate reduction or insufficient fixation.

It can be difficult to judge the extent to which any part of a complex fracture contributes to an unstable joint. Generally, the position of the talus will help to explain the lesions. In an unstable joint, the talus will always be translated:

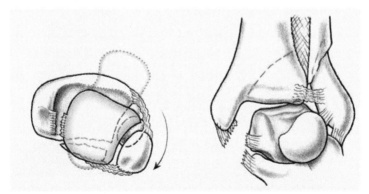

Fig. 3. Posterolateral rotatory malunion. Owing to the posterolateral subluxation of the talus the radiographic appearance simulates lateral joint space narrowing in the anteroposterior view and anterior opening of the ankle in the lateral view. The posterior malleolar fragment may show a fibrous nonunion. The lateral malleolus is rotated externally, shortened, and in valgus (in low fibular fractures).

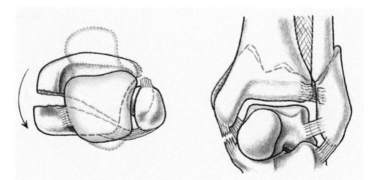

Fig. 4. Posteromedial rotatory malunion. The talus subluxes posteromedially owing to the pull of the intact deep deltoid ligament, which inserts at the displaced posterior half of the medial malleolus. The lateral malleolus is shortened and displaced posteriorly. Usually these deformities represent residual displacement after reduction of a posterior fracture-dislocation.

1. If there is lateral translation of the talus, we will find lesions of the deltoid ligament or the medial malleolus and a malunion of the lateral malleolus (see **Figs. 1** and **2**);
2. If there is posterolateral translation, we will find a ruptured deltoid ligament and a malunion of the lateral and posterior malleolus ("Volkmann's triangle"; see **Fig. 3**); and
3. If there is posteromedial translation, we will find malunion of the lateral malleolus, rupture of the anterior tibiofibular ligament and malunion of the posteromedial corner (see **Fig. 4**).

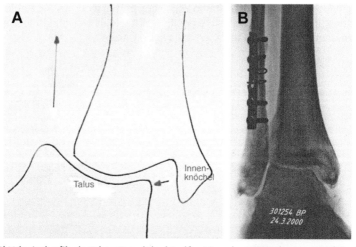

Fig. 5. (*A*) Why is the fibula "short" and the hindfoot in valgus? Displacement of the talus in a lateral direction will result in this deformity because the tibial plafond is not completely, flat but slightly convex. (*B*) Because the lateral ankle ligaments always remain intact in ankle fractures, the anatomic relationships between the lateral malleolus and the talus are not altered, as is well visible in this radiograph. Obvious signs of lateral talar displacement malunion are the increased medial clear space and the widened tibiofibular (syndesmosis) space.

Before any surgical reconstruction is planned, all these pathologic conditions (bone, ligaments, and scarring) have to be assessed.

PREOPERATIVE PLANNING

The assessment of the direction and magnitude of the malunion may be difficult. Certainly, standing radiographs in the standard projections are the key to the diagnosis of malunion. The 3 classic signs or criteria for normal or abnormal fibular length ([1] the lines of the tibial plafond and the surface of the talar dome should be parallel; [2] unbroken "Shenton's" line of the ankle; and [3] unbroken curve between the lateral part of the talar articular surface and the fibular recess) have been described by Weber and Simpson.[2] Other signs as an abnormal talocrural angle and the bimalleolar angle[3] may be of help. Perera and Myerson[4] summarized the radiographic markers of ankle malunion.

Two projections of conventional radiographs are needed: anteroposterior and lateral views, with the patient standing. It is mandatory that these views be performed under load. This will reveal the direction of the subluxation of the talus (lateral, medial, posterolateral, posteromedial) under physiologic conditions. Radiographs of the uninjured side serve as a template for correction.

We advocate performing additional CT scans in all cases. This imaging modality will yield important information about the pathologic morphology of the malunion, bone fragments, and talar position. Three-dimensional image reconstruction will help to understand and plan the reconstructive steps to undertake.

Although diagnosis and the treatment algorithm for malunions is based on radiologic examinations of bony structures, MRI may be of use in unclear situations. It can detect excessive scar tissue formation in syndesmotic injuries and soft tissue interposition as well as cartilage lesions and areas of osteonecrosis. Nevertheless, MRI will not really be of help for the surgical procedure.[5,6]

After the malunion has been documented, a treatment plan has to be drawn up. The plan should address surgical approach, soft tissues (scar removal), osteotomy, correction (angle, interposition of bone, donor site if needed), osteosynthesis, and implants. The technical details of different osteotomies have been published by different authors.[4,7]

The goal of corrective surgery is restoration of the normal ankle anatomy. In terms of stability, this means that the subluxed talus has to be reduced into its normal position. Therefore, all scar tissue and all bony deformities that interfere with repositioning the talus have to be removed or corrected by osteotomy.

PREPARATION AND PATIENT POSITIONING

Standard skin preparation is undertaken. Preoperative antibiotic single shot prophylaxis is administered. The patient is positioned supine, in the lateral decubitus or prone position according to the osteotomies that have to be performed. Generally a thigh tourniquet is used.

SURGICAL APPROACHES

Operations to correct malunions of the ankle include osteotomies of the medial, lateral, and posterior malleolus ("Volkmanns triangle"); the posteromedial corner; or combinations of these procedures. A supramalleolar tibial osteotomy may be required if the alignment of the tibial joint line has been altered (impaction fracture). The surgical approaches should take into account the previous skin incisions. It is important to preserve vascularization of the skin flaps. In cases of excessive scarring or critical soft tissue conditions, it may be helpful to plan the surgery in collaboration with a plastic surgeon.

Medial Malleolus

The previous medial approach is used. If there had been no surgery before at the medial side, we prefer a longitudinal incision.[8] The incision is centered on the tip of the medial malleolus, beginning over the dorsomedial surface of the tibia and is curved anteriorly in direction of the navicular tuberosity. The skin flaps are mobilized, avoiding the greater saphenous vein and the saphenous nerve, which run together anteriorly. A longitudinal incision is made anteriorly in the joint capsule to give view and access to the anterior part of the ankle joint. The flexor retinaculum is incised to identify the tibialis posterior tendon that is, retracted posteriorly. The entire medial malleolus is now exposed.

Lateral Malleolus and Small Posterior Malleolus

The previous lateral approach is used. Usually, this is a longitudinal incision along the posterior margin of the fibula. After reaching the distal end of the lateral malleolus, the incision may be continued for 1 to 2 cm in a slight forward curve. If the incision begins proximal for high fibular malunions, attention is paid to the superficial peroneal nerve.

If a small posterior tibial fragment needs correction, it is approached through the osteotomy of the lateral malleolus. The fibula is cut transversely. The anterior talofibular ligament is divided, and the distal fragment of the lateral malleolus is rotated laterally.

Larger Posterior Malleolus and Posterior Tibial Fragment (Posteromedial Corner)

The patient is positioned prone. A sand bag or cushion is placed under the ankle. This allows extension of the ankle during the operation. The previous approach is used. This is usually a posterolateral longitudinal incision that will now need enlargement proximally. Otherwise, the incision for a posterolateral approach is placed longitudinally, halfway between the posterior border of the lateral malleolus and the lateral border of the Achilles tendon. This gives access to the interval between the peroneal muscles and the flexor hallucis longus muscle. This approach provides the best visualization of the posterior tibial rim. Attention has to be paid to the lesser saphenous vein and the sural nerve that run together. Alternatively, the posteromedial corner of the tibia can be corrected through a (postero-) medial approach (which can be done in a supine position).

OPERATIVE PROCEDURE
Step 1: Medial Malleolus

Malunion of the medial malleolus alone is rare. Mostly the medial malleolus is 1 part of a complex deformity with malunion medially and laterally and/or posteriorly. After exposure of the medial joint space and the groove of the tibialis posterior tendon, the osteotomy is performed in the former fracture plane. In supination/adduction malunions the osteotomy will have a vertical direction. The mobilized fragment is then pushed distally and fixed with a K-wire. In a lateralized medial malleolar malunion, the osteotomy may be more difficult. It will be in a more horizontal direction, and sometimes it may be necessary to perform a dome osteotomy with a curved chisel. After reduction, the fragment is again fixed by a K-wire. Image intensifier control of the reduced talus under the tibial plafond is mandatory. Definitive fixation is obtained by traditional fixation by screws.

In fixed valgus malunion of the fibula, the osteotomy of the lateral malleolus and scar tissue resection, thus allowing the necessary medial translation of the talus, has to be performed before the medial malunion can be reduced (and vice versa).

Step 2: Lateral Malleolus

After exposure of the lateral malleolus, different osteotomies can be performed. The classic horizontal osteotomy[4] (see **Fig. 7**) can be used in almost all slight and severe deformities because it corrects length, rotation, and axial alignment. Nevertheless, interposition grafting will be necessary to achieve solid bone healing at the osteotomy. In a malunion that requires lengthening of 4 to 5 mm and only minimal rotational correction, an oblique or Z-shaped osteotomy[7] may be useful. These techniques do not require bone grafting.

There are often osteophytes (**Fig. 6**) and scar tissue between the fibula and the tibia that have to be excised. Otherwise, lengthening and derotation of the lateral malleolus and medialization of the talus will not be possible. It may be necessary as well to free the widened space between the medial malleolus and the talus from intervening scar tissue (see **Fig. 5**) before anatomic reduction becomes possible. If the medial malleolus has been osteotomized it is fixed at this moment. Then a small fragment plate (2.7 or 3.5 mm AO-LCP [Association of Osteosynthesis-locking compression plate] or similar) is fixed to the lateral malleolus. The malleolus is then maintained in a reduced position by a tension/compression device.

Alternatively, K-wires may be used for temporary fixation after manual translation. Classically, a cortiococancellous graft from the tibial metaphysis[2] (**Fig. 7**) is now placed into the osteotomy to fill the gap. We believe that excised bone from the malunion functions as well. This avoids additional donor site morbidity. Finally, the plate is fixed without compression (**Fig. 8**). If extensive scar removal in the peroneal groove and debridement of the syndesmosis was performed, it may be necessary to additionally stabilize the mortise with a (temporary) syndesmosis screw or K-wires. After irrigation, the wound it is closed with absorbable sutures.

Step 3: Posterior Malleolus and Dorsomedial Corner

The posterior malleolus (**Fig. 9**) can be exposed through the osteotomy of the lateral malleolus. The osteotomy of the posterior malleolus can be done with a chisel directed

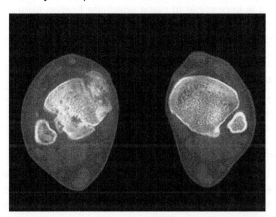

Fig. 6. Computed tomography scans of both ankles, showing the tibiofibular notch. Normal configuration of the ankle on the right side. On the left side, there is diastasis between the fibula and tibia as well as osteophytes on the tibial side. (*From* Weber D, Borisch N, Weber M. Treatment of malunion in ankle fractures. Eur J Trauma Emerg Surg 2010;36:522; with permission.)

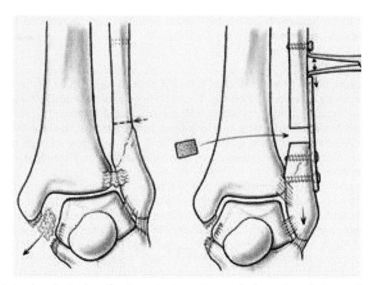

Fig. 7. Lateral malleolar lengthening osteotomy. Removal of scar tissue between the medial malleolus and talus, osteotomy of the fibula, lengthening with distraction device, and grafting. (*From* Weber D, Borisch N, Weber M. Treatment of malunion in ankle fractures. Eur J Trauma Emerg Surg 2010;36:523; with permission.)

from lateral to medial (**Fig. 10**). The direction of the osteotomy is controlled fluoroscopically. It may be safe to use an additional posteromedial approach for better control of the exit of the osteotomy. Fixation of the reduced malleolus can be done with 3.5-mm screws in anteroposterior direction. For internal fixation of the osteotomized and reduced posterior malleolus with an antiglide plate (eg, a 3.5 mm AO [Association of Osteosynthesis]-tubular plate), the posterior tibia is approached through the interval between the flexor hallucis longus and the peroneal muscles (posterolateral approach).

A posteromedial correction[9] may be performed from medially or dorsolaterally. Although the entire posterior tibial rim is well visible from either of these approaches, in our experience it is impossible to place adequate fixation from a single approach into the posteromedial fragment without undue strain to the soft tissues. A bilateral posterior approach, posterolateral and posteromedial, is therefore recommended for this posteromedial pathology.[9]

Immediate Postoperative Care

The ankle is fixed in a plaster cast or comparable splint. Physical therapy may start after wound healing. Active-assisted toe mobilization and lymphatic drainage is recommended. Thromboembolic prophylaxis is started.

Rehabilitation and Recovery

The ankle will be held in a neutral position for 6 weeks. Weight bearing should not be allowed for 6 weeks. Thromboembolic prophylaxis is recommended until full weight bearing is possible. If fixation of the fibulotibial joint (syndesmosis screws) was necessary, the screws should be removed after 8 weeks. After 6 weeks, mobilization of the ankle joint and weight bearing begins. The reconstruction of the ankle mortise is documented radiologically after 6 and 12 weeks in anteroposterior and lateral views. After 12 weeks, the radiographs should be performed under load.

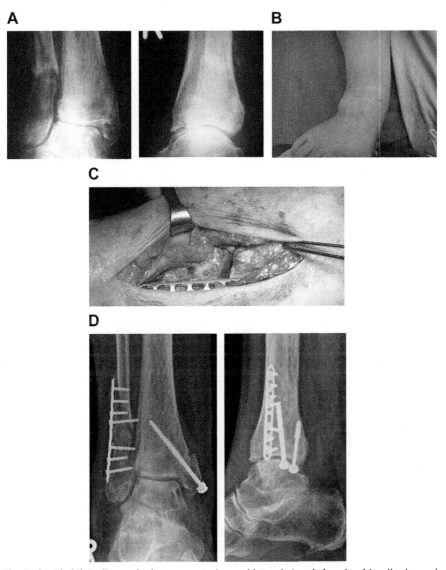

Fig. 8. (*A–D*): (*A*) Radiographs (anteroposterior and lateral views) showing bimalleolar malunion in an 86-year-old female patient 3 months after falling out of bed after total knee replacement surgery. Treatment was strictly functional (no reduction, no fixation). (*B*) Clinical appearance and (*C*) intraoperative image of the right ankle (lateral view). An oblique osteotomy is carried out and the fibula fixed with a dynamic compression plate (2.7 mm AO-ASIF [Association of Osteosynthesis-Association for the study of Internal Fixation]). (*D*) Radiographs 10 days after correction show reduction of the talus and fixation of the medial and lateral malleolus. (*From* Weber D, Borisch N, Weber M. Treatment of malunion in ankle fractures. Eur J Trauma Emerg Surg 2010;36:524; with permission.)

Clinical Results in the Literature

The clinical findings reported in the literature (**Table 1**) are the results of level of evidence IV or V studies. A very detailed literature research has been published by van

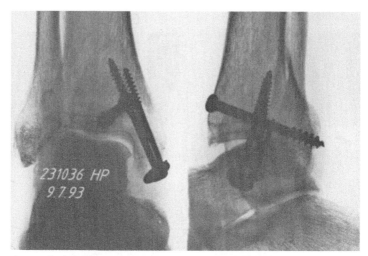

Fig. 9. Radiographs (anteroposterior [AP] and lateral views) showing malunion of the Volkmann triangle and dorsal subluxation of the talus fixed by an AP screw.

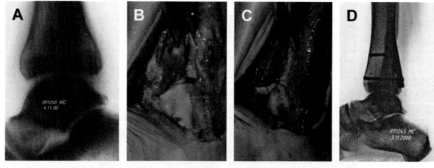

Fig. 10. (*A–D*): (*A*) Radiographic tomography showing malunion of the posterior malleolar fragment. (*B*) Intraoperative findings with proximal dislocation of fragment in the lateral view after osteotomy of the lateral malleolus. (*C*) Intraoperative image showing the osteotomized and reduced posterior malleolus. (*D*) Radiograph (lateral view) at 2 weeks showing the reduced fragment fixed with a 3.5 mm third tubular antiglide plate.

Table 1				
Reported results in the literature after osteotomy for ankle malunion				
Author, Year	**Patients**	**Follow-up (y)**	**Good**	**%**
Yablon & Leach,[11] 1989	26	7	23	88
Weber & Simpson,[2] 1985	23	11	17	74
Weber et al,[18] 2001	8	3.9	6	75
Weber & Ganz,[16] 2003	4	4–6	3	75
El-Rosasy & Ali,[15] 2013	17	2.7	12	67
Reidsma et al,[14] 2010	57	15.5	41	85

Wensen and colleagues[6] in 2009. In almost all studies,[10–18] the mid- and long-term outcomes after correction of malunited malleolar fractures are satisfactory. Good and very good results are reported in 67% to 91% of cases. This means that patients experience an important reduction of pain and a better function in daily activities and often return to their preinjury activity level. A biomechanical study revealed a high accuracy for correction of length (within 1.3 mm) and malrotation (within 1.6°) in the hands of experienced surgeons.[13]

SUMMARY

The goal of reconstructive surgery for a malunited malleolar fracture is restoration of axial alignment and a congruent joint surface to preserve the ankle joint and to avoid progression of degenerative changes already present at the time of correction. Several osteotomies have been described.

Corrective osteotomies for malleolar malunion show good results in more than 70% of patients in the majority of mid- and long-term studies. The existence of arthritic changes before correction of malunion is the major feature that is, associated with poorer clinical and radiologic outcome. Nevertheless patients seem to benefit from a rebalanced ankle for years. Further surgery as arthrodesis or ankle replacement is needed in 10% to 15% of all patients after a follow-up period of 3 to 7 years. Joint-sparing osteotomies are therefore a valid alternative to ankle fusion or replacement especially in young patients with only mild signs of posttraumatic arthritis.

REFERENCES

1. Ramsey PL, Hamilton W. Changes in tibiotalar area of contact caused by lateral talar shift. J Bone Joint Surg Am 1976;58:356–7.
2. Weber BG, Simpson LA. Corrective lengthening osteotomy of the fibula. Clin Orthop Relat Res 1985;199:61–7.
3. Rolfe B, Nordt W, Sallis JG, et al. Assessing fibular length using bimalleolar angular measurements. Foot Ankle 1989;10:104–9.
4. Perera A, Myerson M. Surgical techniques for the reconstruction of malunited ankle fractures. Foot Ankle Clin N Am 2008;13:737–51.
5. Han SH, Lee JW, Kim S, et al. Chronic tibiofibular syndesmosis injury: the diagnostic efficiency of magnetic resonance imaging and comparative analysis of operative treatment. Foot Ankle Int 2007;28:336–42.
6. van Wensen RJA, Bekerom van den MPJ, Marti RK, et al. Reconstructive osteotomy of fibular malunion: review of the literature. Strategies Trauma Limb Reconstr 2011;6:51–7.
7. Weber D, Borisch N, Weber M. Treatment of malunion in ankle fractures. Eur J Trauma Emerg Surg 2010;36:521–4.
8. Hoppenfeld S, deBoer P. Surgical exposures in orthopaedics. The anatomic approach. 4th edition. Philadelphia: Lippincott Williams &Wilkins; 2009. p. 619–40.
9. Weber M. Trimalleolar fractures with impaction of the postero-medial tibial plafond: implications for talar stability. Foot Ankle Int 2004;25:716–27.
10. Sinha A, Sirikonda S, Giotakis N. Fibular lengthening for malunited ankle fractures. Foot Ankle Int 2008;29:1136–40.
11. Yablon IG, Leach RE. Reconstruction of malunited fractures of the lateral malleolus. J Bone Joint Surg Am 1989;71:521–7.
12. Chu A, Weiner L. Distal fibula malunions. J Am Acad Orthop Surg 2009;17: 220–30.

13. Heineck J, Serra A, Haupt C, et al. Accuracy of corrective osteotomies in fibular malunion: a cadaver model. Foot Ankle Int 2009;8:773–7.
14. Reidsma II, Nolte PA, Marti RK, et al. Treatment of malunited fractures of the ankle. J Bone Joint Surg Br 2010;92:66–70.
15. El-Rosasy M, Ali T. Realignment-lengthening osteotomy for malunited distal fibular fracture. Int Orthop 2013;37:1285–90.
16. Weber M, Ganz R. Malunion following trimalleolar fracture with posterolateral subluxation of the talus-reconstruction including the posterior malleolus. Foot Ankle Int 2003;24:338–44.
17. Rammelt S, Marti RK, Zwipp H. Gelenkerhaltende osteotomien fehlverheilter sprunggelenk- und pilonfrakturen. Unfallchirurg 2013;116:789–96.
18. Weber D, Fritschy D, Friederich NF, et al. Osteotomy of the distal fibula for correction of posttraumatic malunion. Classical procedure. Orthop Traumatol 2001;9: 273–83.

Treatment of Nonunions After Malleolar Fractures

Brian M. Capogna, MD, Kenneth A. Egol, MD*

KEYWORDS

- Nonunion • Malleolar • Hypertrophic • Atrophic • Oligotrophic

KEY POINTS

- Malleolar nonunions are a rare entity in orthopedic surgery that can lead to debilitating pain and limited function.
- Preoperative optimization with regard to comorbid medical conditions, such as diabetes, vascular disease, malnutrition, and smoking cessation, is an essential component of the treatment plan.
- Through a multimodal approach, malleolar nonunions are reliably treated with operative fixation leading to good patient outcomes with minimal complications.
- Based on the type of nonunion and other patient risk factors surgeons can use adjuncts, such as bone graft, bone morphogenic proteins (BMP), or bone stimulation.

 Video content accompanies this article at http://www.foot.theclinics.com

INTRODUCTION: NATURE OF THE PROBLEM

There are few focused reviews of nonunions of malleolar ankle fractures. Before the routine practice of open reduction and fixation for these fractures, nonunion following rotational ankle fractures was not uncommon. Mendelsohn[1] in his 1965 review and case series of 253 ankle fractures found a nonunion rate of 4.3%. Two hundred forty-one of these patients underwent closed treatment in a cast or splint. Historically, nonunion rates for malleolar fractures were quoted to be somewhere between 5% and 30%.[2–4]

With the work of the AO (Arbeitsgemeinschaft für Osteosynthesefragen) group and improved indications for the stabilization of displaced fractures of the ankle, the rate of malleolar nonunion has declined significantly. One study found that ankle fracture nonunions comprise 6.8% of all nonunions, whereas others simply remark on their

Dr B.M. Capogna has nothing to disclose. Dr K.A. Egol is a consultant for Exactech, and receives royalties from Exactech, Slack, Inc., and Lippincott. He is a member of the board of directors of the Orthopedic Trauma Association.
Department of Orthopaedic Surgery, Hospital for Joint Diseases, New York University Langone Medical Center, 301 E17th Street, New York, NY 10003, USA
* Corresponding author.
E-mail address: kenneth.egol@nyumc.org

rarity.[5–11] Although rare, nonunion following rotationally unstable ankle fractures can have detrimental effects on patient outcomes leading to continued debilitating pain, instability, and late posttraumatic osteoarthritis.[5,9,12,13]

PATHOPHYSIOLOGY OF NONUNION

Nonunion is complete arrest of the healing process following a fracture.[14] Although several definitions exist, there is generally no evidence of progressive healing on serial radiographs taken over 3 to 6 months. The cause of all nonunions is grouped within one of four categories: (1) those secondary to excessive motion, (2) those caused by vascular insufficiency, (3) those caused by bony gaps, and (4) those secondary to infection. Classically, nonunions are described as hypertrophic, oligotrophic, or atrophic.[15] A hypertrophic nonunion is characterized by abundant callus surrounding the fracture site without bony healing. In this situation there is adequate blood supply and biologic factors for healing, but inadequate stability at the fracture site. Perren and Cordey demonstrated that micromotion at the fracture site leads to increased collagen formation and an inhibitory effect on osteoblasts.[16,17] Perren also described the inter-fragmentary strain theory. Strain is the change in height or length that a material undergoes during loading divided by the original height or length. This theory relates the type of tissue formed to the amount of strain in the environment between healing fracture fragments. Large strains lead to the formation of fibrous granulation tissue, intermediate strains to the formation of cartilaginous tissue, and small strains to the formation of bone by direct healing.

Oligotrophic nonunions do not display an abundant callus as in hypertrophic nonunion. In this situation, there is an intact blood supply to allow for healing. However, nonunion results in the context of distracted fracture fragments, malalignment, inadequate fragment apposition, or improper fixation. Atrophic nonunion results from a lack of blood supply and ability of the body to form the biologic environment necessary for healing. In this scenario callus is minimal or absent. Radiographs show blunted, atrophic, osteopenic fracture ends (**Table 1**).

Risk factors for nonunion can be intrinsic to the patient or extrinsic. Nonunion is more likely to occur if there is insufficient stability, poor reduction, poor blood supply, or interposed soft tissue in the fracture site. Interposed soft tissue can play an important role in malleolar fractures because periosteum or nearby tendons can be partially entrapped between the fragments. Another potential contributor is the effect of the synovial lining and synovial fluid disrupting the fracture hematoma.[1,6] Additionally,

Table 1
Classification of nonunion

Type of Nonunion	Etiology	Radiographs	Treatment
Hypertrophic	Inadequate stability at the fracture site	Abundant callus, persistent fracture line	Primary or revision fixation for added stability
Oligotrophic	Distracted fragments, malalignment, improper fixation	Callus may or may not be present, persistent fracture line	Reduce and stabilize with proper fixation
Atrophic	Inadequate biology, malnutrition, vascular disease, smoking, diabetes mellitus	Callus minimal or absent, fracture ends blunted, persistent fracture line	Primary or revision fixation with addition of bone graft or bone morphogenic protein

several patient factors have been correlated with increasing rates of nonunion including diabetes, tobacco use, obesity, history of radiation therapy, advanced age, and infection.[5,6,8,12,18–20] Thus, treatment of nonunion requires a multimodal approach to control for and minimize these risk factors.

SURGICAL TECHNIQUE
Evaluation

Investigation of a suspected nonunion about the ankle should begin with a complete history, physical examination, radiographs, and routine laboratory examinations. The history should focus on the location and quality of pain, recent or antecedent trauma, previous surgery, onset and timing of symptoms, and presence of fevers. Additionally, the clinician should inquire about a history of diabetes, vascular disease, smoking, or alcohol use. The physical examination may reveal tenderness at the fracture site, persistent swelling, or even grossly mobile segments.

Most malleolar fracture nonunions are clearly evident on plain radiographs as a persistent fracture line with or without surrounding callus depending on the type of nonunion. When plain radiographs are inconclusive, computed tomography (CT) scan is the diagnostic modality of choice with excellent sensitivity and high intraobserver reliability (**Fig. 1**).[21] Single-photon emission CT has limited investigation in the literature. One study showed that it has a low sensitivity but a high specificity for excluding infection and confirms a nonviable fracture environment.[22]

In patients with prior surgery, artifact can limit the investigator's ability to evaluate the fracture site or there may be a contraindication to its use. Nuclear imaging, such as three-phase bone scan, may be useful in these instances, although its use has fallen out of favor with improved CT techniques. Some have advocated use to assess the biologic activity of the fracture site. Niikura and colleagues[23] compared plain radiographs with bone scans in 48 aseptic nonunions and found there was uniform increased uptake in all hypertrophic and more than half of the oligotrophic nonunions. Deficient uptake was seen in 17% of the oligotrophic and 57% of atrophic nonunions limiting the specificity of this modality. When there is uncertainty about the presence of nonunion an alternative modality the surgeon may perform is a dynamic fluoroscopic examination. While applying stress across the suspected nonunion a fluoroscopic image is obtained to confirm gross mobility at the fracture site. This is most useful in cases without prior operative fixation because any implanted hardware can limit the surgeon's ability to detect subtle motion under fluoroscopic imaging.[24]

Several laboratory examinations can help identify the cause of nonunion and aid in treatment. In situations where infection is suspected routine laboratory analysis should be performed. C-reactive protein and erythrocyte sedimentation rate levels are useful screening tools when there is suspicion of an infected nonunion. Rarely, a complete blood count can give clues to the presence of infection with an elevated leukocyte count. In patients with diabetes the hemoglobin A_{1C} can provide important information regarding the patient's long-term glycemic control. Several other serum tests including albumin, prealbumin, transferrin, calcium, and vitamin D levels can indicate patients with poor nutritional status who might benefit from supplementation before and after operative intervention.

Before operative intervention all nonoperative modalities should be exhausted so long as the patient and surgeon are in agreement on the treatment plan. Another modality that can be used before operative intervention is localized patient-administered external bone stimulation. Two options currently exist: low-intensity pulsed ultrasound and electrical stimulation. To date, there are no extensive studies prospectively

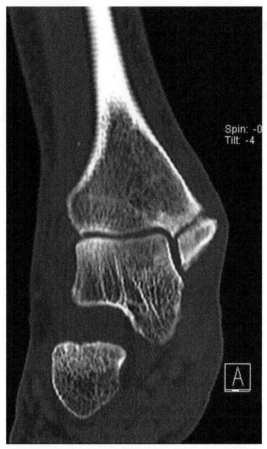

Fig. 1. A 64-year-old man presents for evaluation of continued medial ankle pain 6 months following closed treatment in a cast for an isolated medial malleolus fracture. CT scan confirms medial malleolar nonunion.

analyzing their use in ankle fracture nonunion. Most of the literature focuses on its use in tibial shaft nonunion. These studies often lack adequate power, are nonrandomized, and do not control for the location of nonunion.[25,26] A retrospective study of 71 patients with tibial nonunion showed a healing rate of 73% treated with low-intensity pulsed ultrasound. This was significantly increased when compared with the highest reported rate of spontaneous healing.[27]

Likewise studies of electrical bone stimulation are limited. Sharrard[28] reported increased union rates in patients with delayed union of tibial shaft fractures in a randomized, double-blind, multicenter trial. Another prospective trial of 34 patients with tibial nonunion reported healing in 16 of 18 (89%) in the study arm treated with pulsed electromagnetic stimulation compared with 8 of 16 (50%) of control subjects. The authors did note that the control group had more active smokers than the study arm.[29] Adie and colleagues[30] performed a recent randomized, double-blind, multicenter trial to evaluate pulsed electromagnetic stimulation on patients with acute tibial shaft fractures. They found that, as an adjunct treatment, it did not prevent the need for secondary surgery for either nonunion or delayed union. There was also no difference in time to radiographic union or patient-reported functional outcomes.

Preoperative Planning

Treatment of an ununited fracture begins preoperatively by identifying and controlling extrinsic risk factors for continued failure. This includes tightening glycemic control in coordination with endocrinology, optimizing nutritional status, and enacting a smoking cessation protocol. If serum levels of vitamin D and calcium are low patients can receive supplementation to normalize levels before surgical intervention. In patients with peripheral vascular disease a vascular surgery evaluation is necessary to ensure that a patient does not have a correctable vascular insufficiency. If surgical intervention is indicated, intraoperative cultures should be obtained in all previously operated fractures to evaluate for occult infection. In the case of infected nonunion, treatment should also include prolonged perioperative culture-specific antibiotics and consultation with an infectious disease specialist.

The history, physical examination, and imaging should guide the surgeon as to how to address the nonunion. Generally speaking hypertrophic nonunions lack stability and should be revised with more stable fixation and compression if possible. Oligotrophic nonunions require appropriate reduction and proper fixation. For atrophic nonunions the biologic environment is devoid of factors for healing, thus necessitating addition of osteoconductive and osteoinductive material, such as bone graft, osteopromotors, or bone morphogenic protein (BMP).

Preparation and Patient Positioning

The patient is brought to the operating room and placed on the operating table in the supine position. A tourniquet may be applied to the operative thigh and a bump is placed under the ipsilateral hip to provide internal rotation of the leg (**Fig. 2**). If the surgeon is solely addressing the medial malleolus, no bump is required, because external rotation of the limb facilitates an easier surgical approach (**Fig. 3**). The leg is placed on a radiolucent foam block to allow for easy anteroposterior and lateral imaging. A large or small image intensifier should be available in the room and ready for use. If addressing both medial and lateral malleoli or just the lateral malleolus the fluoroscopic machine is placed on the side opposite the affected limb to facilitate imaging and surgeon positioning. If only the medial malleolus is being addressed, the machine is placed on the same side as the surgical limb so that the surgeon may work from

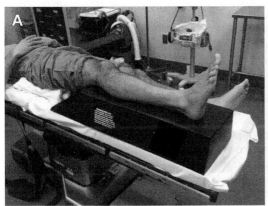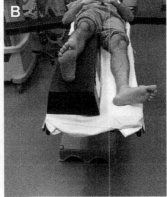

Fig. 2. (*A*) A bump is placed under the operative hip if addressing both the lateral and medial malleoli. (*B*) The patella should be pointed upward to facilitate access to either the lateral or medial side of the limb by the surgeon.

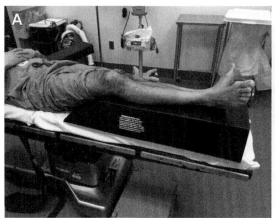 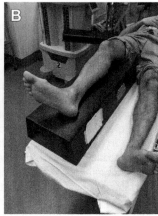

Fig. 3. (A) If only addressing the medial malleolus no bump is required because external rotation of the limb facilitates access to the medial side. (B) The surgeon stands on the opposite side of the limb or foot of the table for the surgical approach.

the foot of the table on the medial side of the limb. If autologous iliac crest bone graft or aspiration is to be performed the donor site should be prepared into the sterile field for simultaneous harvesting.

Surgical Approach

Attention should be focused to any prior surgical incisions. If possible they should be incorporated into the planned incision for fixation of the nonunion. Lateral malleolar fractures are approached from a direct lateral incision centered over the fracture nonunion site. Alternatively, if the surgeon prefers posterolateral plating, the incision is marked along the posterior border of the fibula. The medial malleolus is approached via a direct medial straight or curvilinear incision. During the approach, care should be taken to preserve soft tissue attachments and limit periosteal stripping to maintain vascularity to the fracture fragments. However, this can often be difficult, because stripping is often required to mobilize the fragments for proper reduction. The fracture site is identified and mobilized. All interposed fibrous soft tissue should be removed from the nonunion site with a scalpel or curettes. In atrophic nonunions, a lack of blood supply is addressed by decortication or intramedullary drilling of fracture ends to promote bleeding. The fracture fragments can then be reduced under direct visualization and provisionally held in place with pointed reduction clamps or Kirschner wires before definitive fixation.

Surgical Procedure: Medial Malleolar Nonunion

Most medial malleolar nonunions are addressed by revision of fixation with partially threaded cancellous screws. Distal medial malleolar fractures are assessed by performing an intraoperative stress examination. This can determine if the deep deltoid maintains attachment to a stable portion of the medial malleolus. If a very distal fragment does not contribute to ankle stability but is identified as a source of pain, fragment excision can also be considered.

> Step 1. After identification of the nonunion site a scalpel is used to free soft tissue attachments and mobilize the distal segment. The deltoid attachment should be maintained to protect the blood supply to the fragment.

Step 2. Book-open the fracture site and hold with a dental pick or Freer elevator to aid in removal of fibrous or interposed soft tissue and allow for irrigation. If the fracture ends are atrophic they may be drilled using a 2.0 mm drill bit to induce bleeding.

Step 3. At this point, if indicated, osteopromoting materials or bone graft are added and impacted into the fracture ends before reduction.

Step 4. Once adequate bone graft material has been added, reduce the fracture and provisionally hold with Kirschner wires or pointed reduction clamps. A pilot hole is drilled in the proximal fragment using a 2.0 mm drill bit to allow for easier placement of a pointed reduction clamp.

Step 5. Obtain fluoroscopic images to ensure proper reduction. Once satisfied the surgeon proceeds with fixation of their choice using either cannulated or noncannulated partially threaded cancellous screws to gain compression at the site.

Step 6. Two partially threaded screws are placed, one anterior and one posterior in the medial malleolus. Screws should be parallel to each other and perpendicular to the fracture site to allow for symmetric compression without rotation or translation of the fragment (**Fig. 4**).

Step 7. The wound is irrigated and closed with 2–0 vicryl suture for the subcutaneous layer and 3–0 nylon horizontal mattress sutures for the skin.

Surgical Procedure: Lateral Malleolar Nonunion

Lateral malleolar nonunions can generally be addressed by revision of fixation or primary fixation with a plate and screw construct (**Fig. 5A**). If there is an oblique fracture with flat bony surfaces, lag screw fixation should be performed to provide compression by technique or by design depending on surgeon preference. For very distal avulsion fractures of the lateral malleolus measuring 1 cm or less, fragment excision is considered. This is done in isolation or has been described in coordination with a reconstruction procedure for the lateral ligamentous structures, such as a modified Brostrom.[6,7] The surgeon should assess the ankle under fluoroscopy to ensure that the fragment does not contribute significantly to bony stability before excision. Any and all bony gaps should be addressed with an osteoconductive material, preferably autogenous graft (Video 1).

Step 1. After identification of the nonunion site a scalpel is used to free soft tissue attachments and mobilize the distal segment.

Step 2. Assess for potential interposed soft tissue, such as the peroneal tendons or syndesmotic ligaments.

Step 3. Use external rotation of the ankle and a dental pick to book-open the fracture site and allow for debridement of fibrous tissue followed by irrigation. If the bone ends are atrophic, drilling can be performed to promote bleeding at the fracture site.

Step 4. At this point, if indicated, bone graft or osteopromoting factors are added and impacted into the fracture ends. Reduce the fracture and hold in place with a small lion-jaw or pointed reduction clamp.

Step 5. Obtain fluoroscopic images to assess the reduction and ensure adequate fibular length. Measuring the talocrural angle assesses fibular length. This is the angle subtended by the intermalleolar line and a line perpendicular to the distal tibia articular surface and should measure about 83° (**Fig. 6A**). Alternatively, the radiographic "dime sign" is used as a rough guide for adequate fibular length (**Fig. 6B**).

Step 6. If an oblique fracture line is present, insert a lag screw perpendicular to the fracture site to provide compression of the fragments.

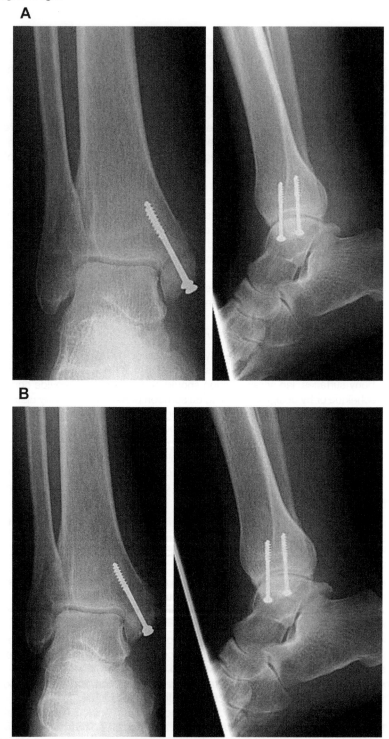

Fig. 4. (*A*) Three-month postoperative radiographs of the patient from **Fig. 1** after fixation with partially threaded cancellous screws and addition of iliac crest bone graft. (*B*) Two-year postoperative radiographs demonstrating complete union of the medial malleolus.

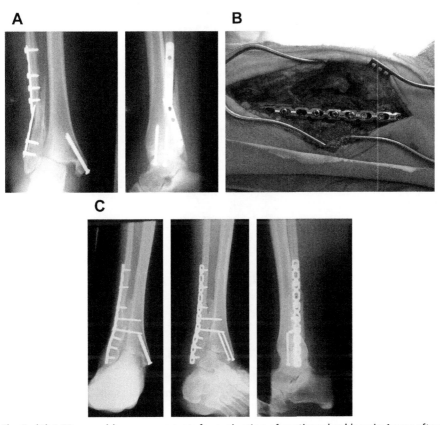

Fig. 5. (*A*) A 71-year-old woman presents for evaluation of continued ankle pain 1 year after open reduction and internal fixation of a bimalleolar ankle fracture. Radiographs demonstrate an atrophic nonunion with failure of her fibular hardware and lateral talar subluxation. (*B*) The patient underwent operative revision with iliac crest bone graft and syndesmotic screw fixation. Pictured is the fibular plate fixation with bone graft bridging the fracture fragments. (*C*) Two-year postoperative radiographs showing complete fracture union. Because of longstanding nonunion the patient had chronic lateral articular surface erosion that resulted in residual valgus postoperatively.

Step 7. Select a plate that provides six cortices of fixation proximally and allows for distal fixation with unicortical screws into the lateral malleolus. A screw hole should be left available for the possibility of syndesmotic screw fixation. Hold the plate to bone manually or with an additional clamp. The plate functions to neutralize and control rotation or is applied in bridge mode in cases of bone loss or fractures not amenable to lag screw compression.

Step 8. Once the plate is fixed to the bone, assess the syndesmosis by performing an external rotation stress examination. If there is syndesmotic instability, one or two syndesmotic screws are inserted about 2 to 3 cm from the joint surface.

Step 9. In cases where the fracture is gapped or there is extensive bone loss, bone graft can be added around the plate taking care to fill all bony gaps (**Fig. 5**B, C).

Step 10. The wound is irrigated and closed in layers. The peroneal fascia is closed with 1–0 vicryl suture and 3–0 nylon horizontal mattress suture is used for skin.

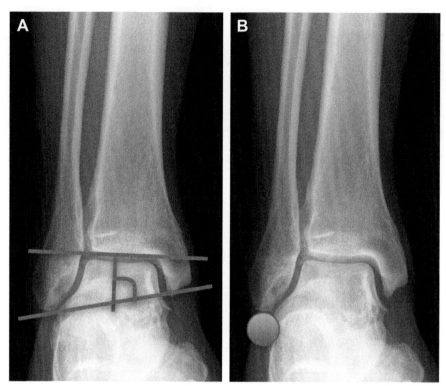

Fig. 6. (A) Radiograph of a normal ankle depicting the talocrural angle. (B) Normal radiographic "dime sign" indicating adequate fibular length.

IMMEDIATE POSTOPERATIVE CARE, REHABILITATION, AND RECOVERY

Postoperatively the patient should be placed in a well-padded short-leg splint and maintain nonweightbearing status. In addition, deep vein thrombosis prophylaxis is our preference. If pain is well controlled, patients may be discharged home on the day of surgery. At the first postoperative visit usually between 10 and 14 days from surgery the splint is removed and the wound assessed. Sutures should be removed at this time and the patient is transitioned to a walking boot. Patients may then begin a passive and active ankle range of motion protocol. Patients should maintain nonweightbearing for a period of 6 weeks at which time radiographs are obtained to evaluate the fracture. If healing is sufficient at 6 weeks, weightbearing in the walking boot is initiated. Patients should be weaned off crutches and the walking boot in the coming weeks until they are full weightbearing at 3 months postoperatively.

SPECIAL CONSIDERATIONS: BONE GRAFTING

Bone graft is useful for patients with atrophic nonunions or bone loss. Cancellous autogenous bone grafting remains the gold standard for the treatment of atrophic non-unions. The principle advantage of autogenous over allograft material is its superior osteoinductive properties. In addition, it provides osteoconductive properties without risk of immunogenicity or disease transfer.[19] Despite these advantages, crushed cancellous bone chips are still a viable alternative or adjunct for management in cases with bone loss and a contraindication to autogenous graft sources. Bone marrow aspirate can also be harvested from the iliac crest and implanted in the area of the fracture nonunion to have an osteoinductive effect. Several other osteoinductive molecules have been studied and shown to have a beneficial effect on healing in animal models. Currently, it is common practice to add BMP to either auto or allograft materials to potentiate their effect. The authors prefer the use of autologous iliac crest bone graft harvested at the time of surgical intervention. We believe that this method provides the fracture site with the best biologic environment for healing.

SPECIAL CONSIDERATIONS: BONE STIMULATION

Bone stimulation therapy is an alternative modality that is considered in the treatment of patients with nonunion about the ankle. The two most commonly used modalities are low-intensity pulsed ultrasound and direct current (DC) bone stimulation. Several in vitro and animal studies have demonstrated a beneficial effect of bone stimulation on osteogenic differentiation and subsequent fracture healing.[31–36] Zhang and colleagues[37] evaluated the effect of DC bone stimulation and BMP-2 on cultured osteoblasts. They found a synergistic effect of DC bone stimulation and BMP-2 with significantly increased cellular metabolic activity, alkaline phosphatase activity, and mineralization. Similarly Koga and colleagues evaluated low-intensity pulse ultrasound and BMP-7 on nonunion tissue harvested from seven patients. They found alkaline phosphatase activity, gene expression levels of alkaline phosphatase and runt-related transcription factor 2, and bone mineralization were higher in the group that received pulse ultrasound plus BMP-7.[38] Despite these results, well-structured randomized comparative clinical trials are lacking in the orthopedic literature.

Implantable DC bone stimulators have been used with success in the treatment of Charcot arthropathy to enhance foot and ankle fusion rates. In these situations the cathode of the bone stimulator is implanted directly into the fracture site. The anode is attached to the battery portion of the stimulator, which is implanted in the extrafascial subcutaneous tissue. Hughes and Anglen[39] evaluated 111 patients who received an implanted bone stimulator for adjunctive treatment of a fracture nonunion. Although not limited to ankle fractures, overall Hughes and Anglen[39] found that 85% of patients healed their nonunion within 7 months of implantation. Complications directly related to the device were three asymptomatic cathode wire breakages and tenderness at the battery site in one patient. Eleven (9.9%) patients developed infection at their fracture site with no infections noted at the battery implantation site. Hockenbury and colleagues[40] reviewed their results of implanted DC stimulation with bone grafting for arthrodesis in 10 patients with Charcot arthropathy of the ankle, hindfoot, or both. They found a fusion rate of 90% at 4 months with minor complications including two superficial infections that resolved with oral antibiotics. Three of the patients required bone stimulator wire removal. It seems that implantable bone stimulation devices may have a beneficial effect on healing in cases of nonunion; however, further prospective randomized trials are required to advocate evidence-based use in these cases.

RESULTS AND OUTCOMES

There are few comparative functional outcomes studies for operatively treated ankle nonunions. It does seem, however, that in the properly selected patient where continued pain is localized to a radiographically confirmed site of nonunion, surgical intervention provides good clinical outcomes. Walsh and DiGiovanni[7] retrospectively reviewed a series of six lateral malleolar nonunions. Operative intervention was performed on five of the patients with the last patient refusing despite persistent symptoms. Union was achieved in all cases with an average time to symptom resolution of 2.3 months. At the time of last follow-up (average, 19.5 months), the authors reported that four of the five patients (80%) had complete resolution of symptoms and the fifth patient had mild persistent lateral discomfort but was self-reported as "90% better."[7]

A study by Khurana and colleagues[6] evaluated 15 patients with malleolar nonunions (12 lateral and 3 medial) that underwent operative fixation. To analyze functional outcomes, the authors compared the study group with a cohort of patients who sustained nonoperative ankle fractures (supination external rotation-2) and a cohort that underwent operative fixation for an unstable ankle fracture (supination external rotation-4). At final follow-up, all cases achieved union (average, 5.2 months). Short Musculoskeletal Functional Assessment scores in the lateral malleolar nonunion group were comparable with those of the SE2 group in the Functional and Daily category, but were worse in the Bothersome, Mobility, and Emotional categories. There were no differences in Short Musculoskeletal Functional Assessment scores between medial malleolar nonunions and any other patient group or between the lateral malleolar group and SE4 patients. A significant difference in postoperative range of motion was seen only when comparing lateral malleolar nonunions with SE2 ankle fractures with limited plantar flexion (27.5° vs 36.1°, respectively). The authors concluded that operative treatment of malleolar nonunions leads to reliable union rates and good functional outcomes with minimal complications.

SUMMARY

Malleolar nonunions are a rare entity in orthopedic surgery. When present, they can lead to debilitating pain and limited function. A thorough preoperative evaluation for any potential causes or risk factors for nonunion is essential. Patients should be preoperatively optimized with regard to comorbid medical conditions, such as diabetes, vascular disease, and malnutrition. Smoking cessation is an essential component of the treatment plan. Based on the type of nonunion and other patient risk factors surgeons can use adjuncts, such as bone graft, BMP, or bone stimulation. Through a multimodal approach, malleolar nonunions are reliably treated with operative fixation leading to good patient outcomes with minimal complications.

SUPPLEMENTARY DATA

Supplementary data related to this article can be found online at http://dx.doi.org/10.1016/j.fcl.2015.09.004.

REFERENCES

1. Mendelsohn HA. Nonunion of malleolar fractures of the ankle. Clin Orthop Relat Res 1965;42:103–18.
2. Banks SW. The treatment of nonunion of fractures of the medial malleolus. J Bone Joint Surg Am 1949;31A:658.
3. Laurent LE. Pseudoarthrosis of the internal malleolus. Ann Chir Gynaecol Fenn 1956;45:48.
4. Mindell ER, Rogers WJ 3rd. Refracture of ununited medial malleolus. Clin Orthopodics 1958;11:233.
5. Chaudhry S, Egol KA. Ankle injuries and fractures in the obese patient. Orthop Clin North Am 2011;42(1):45–53, vi.

6. Khurana S, Karia R, Egol KA. Operative treatment of nonunion following distal fibula and medial malleolar ankle fractures. Foot Ankle Int 2013;34(3):365–71.
7. Walsh EF, DiGiovanni C. Fibular nonunion after closed rotational ankle fracture. Foot Ankle Int 2004;25(7):488–95.
8. Dodson NB, Ross AJ, Mendicino RW, et al. Factors affecting healing of ankle fractures. J Foot Ankle Surg 2013;52(1):2–5.
9. Donken CC, van Laarhoven CJ, Edwards MJ, et al. Misdiagnosis of OTA type B (Weber B) ankle fractures leading to nonunion. J Foot Ankle Surg 2011;50(4):430–3.
10. Myerson MS, Neufeld SK, Uribe J. Fresh-frozen structural allografts in the foot and ankle. J Bone Joint Surg Am 2005;87(1):113–20.
11. King CM, Cobb M, Collman DR, et al. Bicortical fixation of medial malleolar fractures: a review of 23 cases at risk for complicated bone healing. J Foot Ankle Surg 2012;51(1):39–44.
12. Anderson SA, Li X, Franklin P, et al. Ankle fractures in the elderly: initial and long-term outcomes. Foot Ankle Int 2008;29(12):1184–8.
13. Davidovitch RI, Walsh M, Spitzer A, et al. Functional outcome after operatively treated ankle fractures in the elderly. Foot Ankle Int 2009;30(8):728–33.
14. Bucholz R, Court-Brown CM, Heckman JD, et al, editors. Rockwood and Green's fractures in adults. 7th edition. Philadelphia (PA): Lippincott Williams and Wilkins; 2009.
15. Weber BG, Cech O. Pseudarthrosis: pathophysiology, biomechanics, therapy and results. , New York: Grune and Stratton; 1980.
16. Cheal EJ, Mansmann KA, DiGioia AM 3rd, et al. Role of interfragmentary strain in fracture healing: ovine model of a healing osteotomy. J Orthop Res 1991;9(1): 131–42.
17. Lawton DM, Andrew JG, Marsh DR, et al. Mature osteoblasts in human non-union fractures express collagen type III. Mol Pathol 1997;50(4):194–7.
18. Haverstock BD, Mandracchia VJ. Cigarette smoking and bone healing: implications in foot and ankle surgery. J Foot Ankle Surg 1998;37(1):69–74 [discussion: 78].
19. Rodriguez-Merchan EC, Forriol F. Nonunion: general principles and experimental data. Clin Orthop Relat Res 2004;(419):4–12.
20. Egol KA, Tejwani NC, Walsh MG, et al. Predictors of short-term functional outcome following ankle fracture surgery. J Bone Joint Surg Am 2006;88(5):974–9.
21. Bhattacharyya T, Bouchard KA, Phadke A, et al. The accuracy of computed tomography for the diagnosis of tibial nonunion. J Bone Joint Surg Am 2006; 88(4):692–7.
22. Liodakis E, Liodaki E, Krettek C, et al. Can the viability of a nonunion be evaluated using SPECT/CT? A preliminary retrospective study. Technol Health Care 2011; 19:103–8.
23. Niikura T, Lee SY, Sakai Y, et al. Comparison of radiographic appearance and bone scintigraphy in fracture nonunions. Orthopedics 2014;37(1):e44–50.
24. Bishop JA, Palanca AA, Bellino MJ, et al. Assessment of compromised fracture healing. J Am Acad Orthop Surg 2012;20(5):273–82.
25. Jingushi S, Mizuno K, Matsushita T, et al. Low-intensity pulsed ultrasound treatment for postoperative delayed union or nonunion of long bone fractures. J Orthop Sci 2007;12(1):35–41.
26. Nolte PA, van der Krans A, Patka P, et al. Low-intensity pulsed ultrasound in the treatment of nonunions. J Trauma 2001;51(4):693–702 [discussion: 702–3].
27. Rutten S, Nolte PA, Guit GL, et al. Use of low-intensity pulsed ultrasound for post-traumatic nonunions of the tibia: a review of patients treated in the Netherlands. J Trauma 2007;62(4):902–8.

28. Sharrard WJ. A double-blind trial of pulsed electromagnetic fields for delayed union of tibial fractures. J Bone Joint Surg Br 1990;72(3):347–55.
29. Simonis RB, Parnell EJ, Ray PS, et al. Electrical treatment of tibial non-union: a prospective, randomised, double-blind trial. Injury 2003;34(5):357–62.
30. Adie S, Harris IA, Naylor JM, et al. Pulsed electromagnetic field stimulation for acute tibial shaft fractures: a multicenter, double-blind, randomized trial. J Bone Joint Surg Am 2011;93(17):1569–76.
31. Lau JT, Stamatis ED, Myerson MS, et al. Implantable direct-current bone stimulators in high-risk and revision foot and ankle surgery: a retrospective analysis with outcome assessment. Am J Orthop (Belle Mead NJ) 2007;36(7):354–7.
32. Kim IS, Song JK, Song YM, et al. Novel effect of biphasic electric current on in vitro osteogenesis and cytokine production in human mesenchymal stromal cells. Tissue Eng Part A 2009;15(9):2411–22.
33. Kim IS, Song JK, Zhang YL, et al. Biphasic electric current stimulates proliferation and induces VEGF production in osteoblasts. Biochim Biophys Acta 2006; 1763(9):907–16.
34. Yen-Patton GP, Patton WF, Beer DM, et al. Endothelial cell response to pulsed electromagnetic fields: stimulation of growth rate and angiogenesis in vitro. J Cell Physiol 1988;134(1):37–46.
35. Coman M, Hîncu M, Surlin P, et al. Comparative histomorphometric study of bone tissue synthesized after electric and ultrasound stimulation. Rom J Morphol Embryol 2011;52(Suppl 1):455–8.
36. Mollon B, da Silva V, Busse JW, et al. Electrical stimulation for long-bone fracture-healing: a meta-analysis of randomized controlled trials. J Bone Joint Surg Am 2008;90(11):2322–30.
37. Zhang J, Neoh KG, Hu X, et al. Combined effects of direct current stimulation and immobilized BMP-2 for enhancement of osteogenesis. Biotechnol Bioeng 2013; 110(5):1466–75.
38. Lee SY, Koh A, Niikura T, et al. Low-intensity pulsed ultrasound enhances BMP-7-induced osteogenic differentiation of human fracture hematoma-derived progenitor cells in vitro. J Orthop Trauma 2013;27(1):29–33.
39. Hughes MS, Anglen JO. The use of implantable bone stimulators in nonunion treatment. Orthopedics 2010;33(3).
40. Hockenbury RT, Gruttadauria M, McKinney I. Use of implantable bone growth stimulation in Charcot ankle arthrodesis. Foot Ankle Int 2007;28(9):971–6.

Intra-articular Osteotomy for Correction of Malunions and Nonunions of the Tibial Pilon

CrossMark

Stefan Rammelt, MD, PhD*, Hans Zwipp, MD, PhD

KEYWORDS

- Tibial pilon • Fracture • Malunion • Nonunion • Correction • Osteotomy
- Intra-articular • Supramalleolar

KEY POINTS

- Malunions after tibial pilon fractures lead to painful malfunction of the ankle joint and rapidly progress to posttraumatic arthritis.
- Nonunions may result from faulty operative technique or focal necrosis at the distal tibial metaphysis.
- Most malunions and nonunions of the tibial pilon can be salvaged by corrective ankle fusion.
- Joint-preserving corrective osteotomies may be pursued in selected active, compliant patients with good bone stock and cartilage quality at the time of presentation.
- Both intra-articular and supramalleolar deformities have to be corrected in the same setting.

INTRODUCTION

Fractures of the tibial pilon are severe injuries with complex fracture patterns and significant associated articular cartilage and soft tissue damage. The treatment of pilon fractures is challenging, and functional deficits are likely to remain even with perfect anatomic reduction.[1,2]

Most pilon fractures result from high-energy injuries with axial loading like motor vehicle accidents and fall form a height typically involving some degree of

The authors have nothing to disclose.
Foot and Ankle Section, University Center for Orthopaedics & Traumatology, University Hospital Carl Gustav Carus at the TU Dresden, Fetscherstrasse 74, Dresden 01307, Germany
* Corresponding author.
E-mail address: strammelt@hotmail.com

Foot Ankle Clin N Am 21 (2016) 63–76
http://dx.doi.org/10.1016/j.fcl.2015.09.008
foot.theclinics.com

impaction of the metaphyseal bone often with fragmentation and severe damage to the joint surface. The primary cartilage damage caused by axial forces predisposes to the development of posttraumatic arthritis and is a potential source of poor outcomes despite anatomic joint reconstruction.[3,4] Murray and colleagues[5] showed chondrocyte death in all 6 histologic samples taken from comminuted fragments of tibial plafond fractures. Several investigators have noted a close correlation between fracture type and associated complications with signs of posttraumatic arthritis seen in up to 68%.[3,6,7] After Rüedi type 3 and AO/ Orthopaedic Trauma Association type C fractures some radiographic changes of the joint space can be observed in nearly all patients regardless of the kind of treatment.[6] However, arthritis that is detected radiographically does not necessarily become symptomatic, and arthrodesis of the ankle is required in only a small percentage of these cases. The reported rates of secondary ankle fusion range between 1% and 9% after staged open reduction and internal fixation in recent studies.[4,8–10]

Malunions of the tibial plafond, that is, the articular surface of the distal tibia, will lead to eccentric loading of the ankle joint and add to the cartilage wear induced by the injury mechanism. As with other intra-articular fractures, residual steps on the articular joint surface caused by imperfect reduction are a negative prognostic factor, as has been shown in several studies.[8,10,11] In a retrospective review of 113 patients, Kilian and colleagues[12] saw only poor and fair functional results after sole treatment of AO type C pilon fractures with external fixation and related this to improper joint reduction.

Recent studies found higher rates of posttraumatic arthritis, nonunion, and, above all, malunion after external fixation compared with open reduction and internal fixation.[4,13,14] Papadokostakis and colleagues,[15] in a systematic review, found 15 articles referencing 465 pilon fractures treated with external fixation. Malunions were more frequent in ankle-spanning frames (13.4%) than in ankle-sparing frames (5.7%). The same was observed with respect to nonunions, which were reported in 6% and 5%, respectively. It appears that anatomic reduction cannot be achieved with external fixation alone in complex fractures, and secondary dislocation can occur after limited internal fixation.

In addition to intra-articular malunions owing to residual steps and gaps, improper reduction of the metaphyseal area in comminuted pilon fractures lead to supramalleolar axial deviation.[16] These deformities have to be addressed simultaneously during corrective surgery.

INDICATIONS/CONTRAINDICATIONS

Because of the initial cartilage damage at the time of injury and the early onset of symptomatic posttraumatic arthritis in the presence of malunions and nonunions after tibial pilon fractures, only a small percentage of patients will be amenable to joint-preserving corrections.[16]

Intra-articular deformities may be subject to corrective osteotomies along the former fracture planes in the following cases:

- Young, active patients
- Good bone stock
- Sufficient cartilage cover over the weight-bearing areas (first- to second-degree chondromalacia)
- Good compliance with the postoperative protocol to regain a maximum of residual ankle function

Contraindications to joint-preserving osteotomies include:

- Symptomatic posttraumatic arthritis with loss of cartilage over the weight-bearing areas
- Poor bone quality with extensile avascular necrosis (AVN) of the epiphyseal portion of the tibial pilon
- Chronic soft tissue or bone infection
- Poor patient compliance (smoking, substance abuse, severe mental impairment)
- Relevant comorbidities (poorly controlled diabetes mellitus, stage IIb peripheral vascular disease, systemic immune deficiency)

In case of contraindications to joint-preserving osteotomies, corrective fusion of the ankle joint is a viable treatment alternative and will lead to substantial reduction of pain, correction of the deformity, and functional rehabilitation.[17] In the absence of extensile AVN of the distal tibia and good residual motion, total ankle arthroplasty might also be considered. In case of progressive ankle arthritis despite corrective osteotomy, ankle fusion or replacement may be carried out as a secondary procedure on a well-aligned ankle.[18]

SURGICAL TECHNIQUE
Preoperative Planning

Patients with malunions and nonunions after tibial pilon fractures are evaluated clinically with respect to pain, shoe wear, gross deformity, callosities, neurovascular status, residual range of motion, and stability at the ankle joint. The soft tissue conditions around the ankle and hindfoot are of special interest. Pre-existing scars from open wounds, previous approaches, and skin defects have to be respected when planning corrective procedures. Important patient-related factors to be considered are activity level, professional demands, comorbidities (above all osteoporosis, diabetes, and any neurovascular deficits), substance abuse, and inability to comply with the postoperative protocol.

Overall alignment and stability of the ankle is assessed with bilateral weight-bearing anteroposterior and lateral radiographs (**Fig. 1**) supplemented by a hindfoot alignment view. In addition, computed tomographic (CT) scanning is mandatory for determining the exact 3-dimensional outline of the malunion, the position and amount of steps and gaps in the joint surface, and the extent of posttraumatic arthritis and bony union (**Fig. 2**). MRI may be useful to determine the presence and extent of AVN within the tibial plafond or distal metaphysis, osteochondral defects, and associated soft-tissue pathologies like tendon impingement. An ongoing infection should be ruled out with routine leukocyte counts and C-reactive protein serum levels.

Because of the primary cartilage damage at the time of injury and the detrimental effects of intra-articular and extra-articular malalignment on the ankle joint, some radiographic evidence of posttraumatic arthritis will almost invariably be present at the time of correction.[18] The definite decision to preserve or fuse the ankle joint, therefore, is frequently made during reconstructive surgery by visually assessing and directly probing the cartilage quality over the tibial plafond and talus. If a cartilage cover of reasonable quality is present over the weight-bearing areas at the time of correction (ie, no more than second-degree chondromalacia), a joint-sparing osteotomy may be carried out. Both treatment options—corrective ankle fusion and joint reconstruction—and possible consequences must be discussed with the patient before surgery.

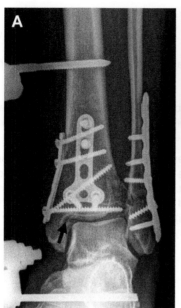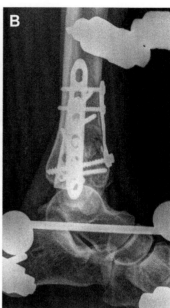

Fig. 1. (*A, B*) Radiographs of a 22-year-old female patient presenting for a second opinion more than 4 weeks after a snowboarding injury. The pilon fracture had been fixed acutely (without preoperative CT scanning) via 3 approaches (central, medial, and lateral). An external fixator is still in place. The images show a lateral shift of the talus and widening of the ankle mortise. A double contour is seen at the medial malleolus (*arrow* in *A*). The articular surface of the distal tibia cannot be assessed reliably.

Surgical Approaches and Patient Positioning

Anatomic corrections of malunions and nonunions of tibial pilon fractures are carried out via the same surgical approaches that would be used in acute fractures.[1,2,19,20] If possible, existing scars from previous surgery are used again, especially if surgical implants have to be removed before correction. Most pilon malunions may be visualized adequately via an anteromedial, central, or anterolateral approach that lies over the entrance (or "trap door") to the former fracture as assessed preoperatively with CT scanning.[21] To gain access to the tibial plafond, an additional medial malleolar osteotomy may be necessary (see **Fig. 8**). For the anterior approaches, the patient is placed in a supine position with a bump placed beneath the ipsilateral hip to place the foot in a neutral position.

In cases of malunions or nonunions after displaced posterior pilon fractures, a posterolateral or, rarely, a posteromedial approach is needed for adequate access and stabilization.[18,22] For these approaches, the patient is placed prone. Rarely, both anterior and posterior approaches are needed. In these cases, corrective surgery may be carried out in a staged manner as suggested for selected acute factures[19] or with intraoperative repositioning of the patient.

SURGICAL PROCEDURES
Anterior Approach

A straight anteromedial, central, or anterolateral incision is carried out over the entrance (trap door) to the former fracture as assessed with preoperative CT scanning

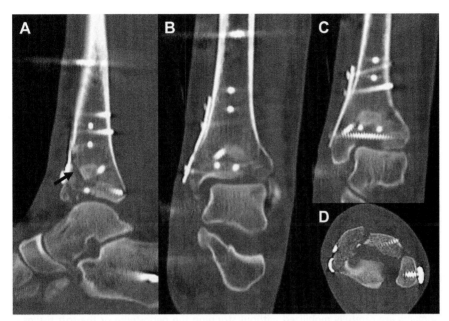

Fig. 2. (*A*) CT scan at 5 weeks shows a solid malunion of the central (die punch) articular fragment that is grossly displaced proximally and tilted (*arrow* in *A*). (*B*) Because of a dehiscence between the anterolateral and anteromedial fragments, the ankle mortise is widened and the talus shifted laterally. (*C, D*) The displaced die punch fragment leaves a large gap in the articular surface of the tibial plafond.

(**Fig. 3**A). The incision may be slightly curved in its distal extension over the talus. With additional supramalleolar malalignment, the incision must extend more proximally to allow adequate mobilization and fixation of the metaphyseal fragment. The scarred anterior joint capsule is resected, and the tibial plafond and talar dome are exposed. Extensive soft tissue or periosteal stripping has to be avoided so as not to jeopardize the delicate blood supply to both the bone and soft tissues. Special care has to be taken not to injure the anterior perforating branch of the fibular artery that constantly penetrates the tibiofibular interosseous membrane about 5 cm above the ankle joint and runs distally across the anterior tibiofibular ligament of the tibiofibular syndesmosis.[1] Therefore, soft tissue or periosteal detachment at the lateral border of the distal tibia and the capsule from the Tubercule de Chaput (Chaput's tubercle) should be avoided.

The anteromedial and anterolateral fragments (Chaput's tubercle) are separated from each other to gain access to the malunited central or posterior fragments (**Fig. 3**B). This may require a first osteotomy depending on the distance between those fragments and the time from injury. The fragments are carefully mobilized without stripping the periosteum or the soft tissues at their margins. Then the malunited central (die punch) fragment is identified and the cartilage quality is assessed by direct probing. Any small, loose, and nonviable fragments are excised. Smaller cartilage defects in the tibia and talus may be subjected to microfracturing. An osteotomy between the die punch fragment and the distal metaphysis is then carried out stepwise and carefully with small chisels under direct vision. Depending on the original fracture anatomy, further osteotomies between the anteromedial and posteromedial or posterolateral and posteromedial fragments have to be carried out. In case of nonunion, the fibrous

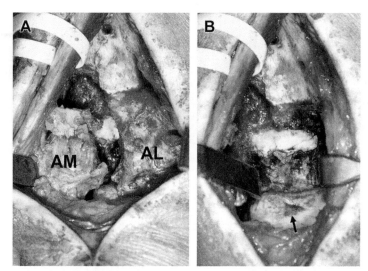

Fig. 3. (*A*) Intraoperative aspect of the distal tibial metaphysis at the site of the trap door shows a wide gap between the anterolateral (Chaput, AL) and anteromedial (AM) fragments 6 weeks after the injury and 10 days after removal of the external fixator. (*B*) The fragments are carefully mobilized without stripping the periosteum or the soft tissues at their margins, revealing the depressed and tilted die punch fragment that carries a complete cartilage cover. Note the corresponding cartilage defect in the central, non–weight-bearing area of the talar dome (*arrow* in *B*). Reduction of the tibial plafond requires an osteotomy of the die punch fragment and between the anteromedial and posteromedial fragments that are both solidly healed at the time of correction. Osteotomy is carried out step wise with small chisels under direct vision.

pseudoarthrosis is resected, and the adjacent cancellous bone debrided from sclerotic or necrotic tissue.[16,18] If the fibula has healed in malalignment, an additional fibular osteotomy is carried out to allow free manipulation of the distal tibial fragments.

After mobilization of the malunited or pseudoarthrotic fragments, correction of the tibial plafond is carried out from posterior to anterior as in acute fractures. A femoral distractor between the tibial shaft and the calcaneus (or talus) is most useful for direct visualization of the tibial joint surface. The reduced fragments are held temporarily with K-wires. In case of multiple fragmentation, transfixation of the fragments is achieved step wise with K-wires that are sharpened on both ends, then introduced from anterior, and pulled out posteriorly until they are flush with the anterior rim of the fragments (**Fig. 4**). Then, the anterolateral and anteromedial fragments are flipped back over the reconstructed joint, thus, closing the trap door and held with a pointed reduction clamp and additional K-wires. The K-wires that have been pulled out posteriorly are now driven back anteriorly to hold the whole joint surface. Anatomic reduction is verified with direct assessment of the joint surface under distraction and fluoroscopically.

Stable internal fixation of the distal tibia is achieved with an interlocking plate connecting the realigned articular portion to the tibial metaphysis (**Fig. 5**). Separate screws or additional plates are introduced according to the individual fracture pattern to reliably stabilize the articular fragments. One or 2 of the introduced K-wires may be cut flush with the anterior tibial rim and left as lost K wires to enhance fixation of the articular fragments. Larger defects resulting from debridement of nonunions and nonviable bone are filled with cancellous bone graft from the proximal tibia or the iliac

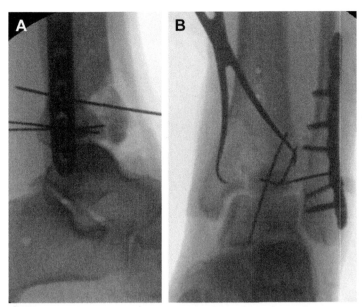

Fig. 4. (*A*) Correction of the plafond is carried out from posterior to anterior after osteotomy of the posterior and die punch fragments. The reduced fragments are held temporarily
with K-wires that are introduced from anterior and pulled out posteriorly until they are
flush with the anterior rim of the fragments. Then, the anterolateral (Chaput) fragment is
flipped back over the reconstructed joint and held with another K-wire. (*B*) Finally, the osteotomized anteromedial fragment is realigned with the anterolateral fragment and the
trap door closed. An additional osteotomy of the fibula is not needed.

crest. The plate must be long enough to achieve adequate stabilization to the tibial
shaft. Longer plates are slid in subcutaneously, and the proximal screws are inserted
percutaneously to minimize additional soft tissue compromise (**Fig. 6**).

Medial Malleolar Osteotomy

Considerable shortening of the medial malleolus (**Fig. 7**) requires a separate lengthening osteotomy to reestablish the ankle mortise and correct varus deformity. In addition, assessment of the intra-articular step-off maybe achieved through the medial
malleolar osteotomy and the intra-articular osteotomy then carried out under direct
vision and fluoroscopic control (**Fig. 8**). The articular fragments are reduced and fixed
with screws through the medial malleolar osteotomy. The medial malleolar fragment is
then shifted distally. After anatomic correction is confirmed fluoroscopically, fixation is
achieved with an interlocking plate.

Supramalleolar Deformity

Any supramalleolar deformity is corrected in the same session by an additional
supramalleolar osteotomy.[16] Because most posttraumatic deformities after pilon
fractures are accompanied by shortening of the distal tibia (see **Fig. 7**), an opening
wedge osteotomy is the treatment of choice provided there are adequate soft tissue
conditions. The osteotomy site is marked with K-wire(s). In the author's preference, a
tricortical bone graft from the iliac crest is used to fill the osteotomy gap (see
Fig. 8C).

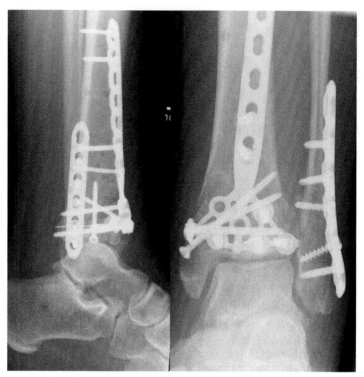

Fig. 5. Postoperative radiographs after fixation of the tibial pilon with an interlocking plate show realignment of the mortise and the tibial metaphysis.

Posterior Approach

Isolated malunions of the posterior tibial rim are best addressed via a posterolateral or posteromedial approach according to the exact fracture anatomy. Fractures of the posterior tibia without disruption of the anterior plafond are rather part of malleolar fractures than pilon fractures.[18,22] However, fractures that involve a considerable portion of the posterior plafond including intercalary depressed fragments are sometimes referred to as *posterior pilon fractures*.[23] So far, distinction between posterior malleolar and posterior pilon fractures is merely a matter of convention. Bartoníček and colleagues[24] recommended the term *posterior pilon fractures* for those involving more than half of the fibular notch. In our experience, only simple, 2-part fractures of the posterior tibial plafond with still intact cartilage are amenable for anatomic reconstruction by corrective osteotomy.

The authors prefer the posterolateral approach, which allows a good exposure over the whole posterior tibia without jeopardizing the medial neurovascular bundle.[18] However, for specific fracture patterns involving the medial part of the posterior tibia, a posteromedial approach either alone or in addition to the posterolateral approach may be useful.[22] The longitudinal incision lies lateral to the Achilles tendon. When dissecting the subcutaneous tissue, care is taken not to injure the sural nerve that crosses from medial to lateral in the proximal part of the incision. The superficial and deep tascia are incised and the flexor hallucis longus muscle and tendon are retracted medially, thus, protecting the posterior neurovascular bundle. Adhesions of the muscle,

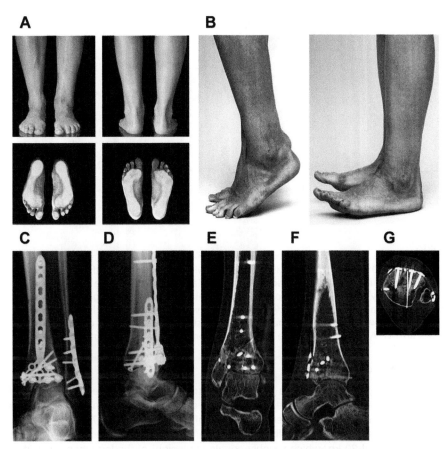

Fig. 6. (*A*, *B*) Clinical aspect of the patient 2 years after correction. The ankle is well aligned with only a small residual edema. Scar formation is limited because of the subcutaneous (less invasive) introduction of the upper limb of the tibial plate. Dorsiflexion of the ankle is slightly limited compared with the formerly uninjured side. (*C*, *D*) Standing radiographs 2 years after corrective osteotomy. (*E–G*) CT scans show anatomic reconstruction of the tibial plafond but also symmetric narrowing of the radiographic joint space suggesting posttraumatic arthritis. The patient so far has little pain but may need an ankle arthrodesis or replacement in the long term (same patient as in **Figs. 1–5**).

tendon, or posterior capsule are resected. Similar to malunions of the posterior talar body, the use of a tibiocalcaneal femoral distractor is most useful to obtain a complete overview over the distal tibial plafond from posteriorly.

Small loose fragments without cartilage cover are excised. The former fracture line is identified and marked with a K-wire. The exact position of the wire is verified with a lateral fluoroscopic view. The lower leg is rotated until the former fracture plane can be clearly delineated. An osteotome is introduced parallel to the K-wire, and osteotomy is carried out from proximal to distal into the tibial plafond. In case of a fibrous nonunion, it is resected and the boney surfaces are debrided until viable bone becomes visible. The posterior fragment is then reduced, and anatomic reduction of the joint surface is confirmed clinically (with distraction) and fluoroscopically. Fragment fixation is achieved with either screws or a posterior antiglide plate.

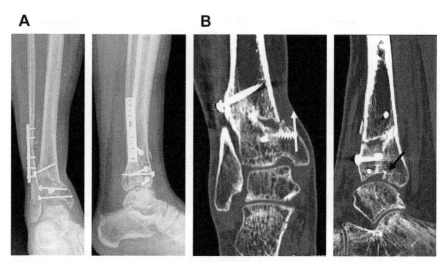

Fig. 7. (*A*) A 30-year-old female patient presents with ongoing pain and inability to walk 6 months after minimally invasive screw fixation of a tibial pilon fracture. The standing radiographs show a varus deformity of the distal tibial metaphysis and irregularity within the tibial joint surface. (*B*) CT scan shows an additional vertical malunion of the medial malleolus (*white arrow*) intra-articular malunion with a step off in the tibial plafond of 5 mm (*black arrow*). A metaphyseal bone defect is seen on the medial aspect of the distal tibia.

Postoperative Care

Postoperatively, the lower leg is put into a splint or split below-knee cast. Physical therapy with active and passive ankle motion starts on the second postoperative day to maintain motion and prevent recurrence of adhesions. At 5 to 7 days, a walking cast, special boot, or walker is fitted, and patients are mobilized with partial weight bearing of about 20 kg, which roughly equals the weight of the leg when it is put to the ground but not loaded. Depending on the individual bone quality, the amount of bone grafting, and the type of fixation, weight bearing is restricted for 8 to 12 weeks postoperatively. After obtaining weight-bearing radiographs showing full boney union, an active rehabilitation program is started to regain a maximum function for the patient (**Fig. 9**). Prominent implants may be removed after 1 year. For recurrent adhesions or osteophytes resulting in restricted ankle range of motion (mostly dorsiflexion), removal of the implants may be combined with arthrolysis of the ankle joint (**Fig. 10**).

CLINICAL RESULTS IN THE LITERATURE

Early attempts at reconstructive surgery for malunited pilon fractures were fraught with an 80% failure rate.[25] Until recently, there were only a few anecdotal case reports on joint-preserving osteotomies for tibial pilon malunions and nonunions without a detailed follow-up.[26–29]

The only available series in the literature summarized the experience from 2 centers (Amsterdam, Netherlands and Dresden, Germany).[16] Over 21 years, we have treated 14 patients (12 men, 2 women) age 28 to 50 years with corrective intra-articular osteotomy and secondary reconstruction for malunited pilon fractures. The patients presented at an average of 3 months (range, 1–17 months) after the injury. Of these, 3 initially had suffered an AO type B3, 2 an AO type C1, 4 an AO type C2, and 5 an AO type C3 fracture. At the time of presentation, all fractures had already solidly

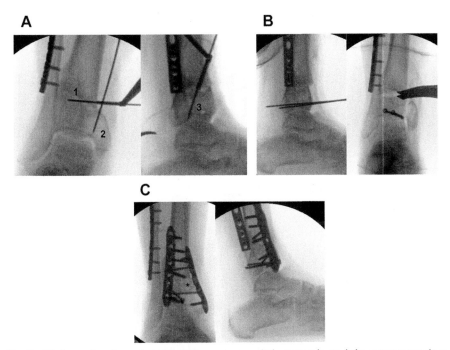

Fig. 8. (*A*) Correction is carried out via an anteromedial approach, and the osteotomy sites are marked with K-wires. The first osteotomy (1) addresses the supramalleolar varus deformity and the second osteotomy (2) the shortened medial malleolus. The intra-articular step off is visualized through the medial malleolar osteotomy, and the intra-articular osteotomy (3) is carried out under direct vision and fluoroscopic control. (*B*) First, the articular fragments are reduced and fixed with screws. Then, the supramalleolar deformity is corrected with an opening wedge and tricortical bone graft from the iliac crest (*asterisk* in C). Finally, the medial malleolar fragment is shifted distally. (*C*) After anatomic correction is confirmed fluoroscopically, the distal tibia is fixed with 2 interlocking plates. The anterolateral plate is slid in subcutaneously through a small anterolateral approach and the proximal screws inserted percutaneously.

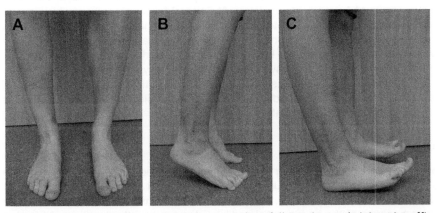

Fig. 9. (*A*) At 2.5 years' follow-up the patient is working full time in an administrative office and reports some pain and swelling after 8 hours of standing and sitting. (*B, C*) On clinical examination, she has a 10° limitation of plantar flexion and a 5° limitation of dorsiflexion.

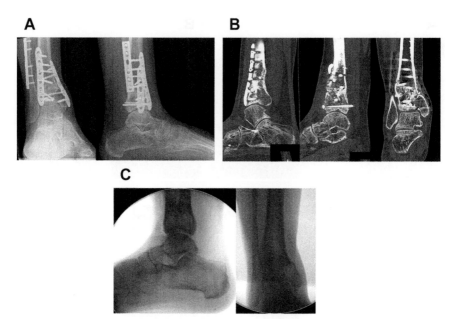

Fig. 10. (*A*) Standing radiographs and (*B*) CT scans show bony union, axial realignment, and full restoration of ankle joint congruity with a 2-mm gap at the site of the intra-articular osteotomy. (*C*) Fluoroscopic images after removal of all implants and arthrolysis of the ankle show anatomic extra- and intra-articular alignment, and intraoperative assessment found a still viable cartilage cover (same patient as in **Figs. 7–9**).

healed in malposition. Three of these patients had an additional focal nonunion or necrosis at the distal tibial metaphysis.

All patients were followed up for an average of 5 years (range, 0.5–10 years). No severe postoperative complications such as hematoma or infections were seen. Late revision surgery was needed for nonunion in 1 case and avascular necrosis of the medial tibial metaphysis in another case. Both were treated with bone grafting and healed uneventfully in the further course. Three patients underwent hardware removal at a minimum of 1 year postoperatively. At 5 years' follow-up, radiographic signs of posttraumatic arthritis were noted in all cases. The clinical result was excellent in one, good in 9, fair in 2, and poor in 2 patients. A late ankle fusion was performed for symptomatic arthritis in the latter 2 patients at 2 and 2.5 years after correction. One patient underwent osteophyte resection and arthrolysis at the ankle joint.

Overall, a surgical revision was performed in 7 of 14 patients (50%), but only 2 of 14 patients (14%) needed a secondary arthrodesis. The subjective clinical outcome was good to excellent in 10 of 14 patients (71%).

SUMMARY

Malunions and nonunions after tibial pilon fractures regularly lead to progressive development of painful posttraumatic ankle arthritis and malposition of the hindfoot with severe functional disability. Most of these conditions will need corrective ankle fusion because of the severe initial cartilage damage and the rapid progression of posttraumatic arthritis with any malposition of the tibial plafond. Joint-preserving correction with secondary anatomic reconstruction is possible in carefully selected patients with intact cartilage, sufficient bone quality, residual function, and good compliance. Osteotomies of solid malunions are planned with preoperative CT scanning. Bone grafting is needed after resection of a fibrous nonunion or sclerotic or necrotic bone. Anatomic reconstruction of malunited tibial pilon fractures may be a viable treatment option especially in young, active patients.

REFERENCES

1. Cronier P, Steiger V, Rammelt S. Early open reduction and internal fixation of pilon fractures. FussSprungg 2012;10(1):12–26.
2. Assal M, Ray A, Stern R. Strategies for surgical approaches in open reduction internal fixation of pilon fractures. J Orthop Trauma 2015;29(2):69–79.
3. Lee YS, Chen SW, Chen SH, et al. Stabilisation of the fractured fibula plays an important role in the treatment of pilon fractures: a retrospective comparison of fibular fixation methods. Int Orthop 2009;33(3):695–9.
4. Wang C, Li Y, Huang L, et al. Comparison of two-staged ORIF and limited internal fixation with external fixator for closed tibial plafond fractures. Arch Orthop Trauma Surg 2010;130(10):1289–97.
5. Murray MM, Zurakowski D, Vrahas MS. The death of articular chondrocytes after intra-articular fracture in humans. J Trauma 2004;56(1):128–31.
6. Wyrsch B, McFerran MA, McAndrew M, et al. Operative treatment of fractures of the tibial plafond. A randomized, prospective study [see comments]. J Bone Joint Surg Am 1996;78(11):1646–57.
7. Pollak AN, McCarthy ML, Bess RS, et al. Outcomes after treatment of high-energy tibial plafond fractures. J Bone Joint Surg Am 2003;85-A(10):1893–900.
8. Patterson MJ, Cole JD. Two-staged delayed open reduction and internal fixation of severe pilon fractures. J Orthop Trauma 1999;13(2):85–91.
9. Boraiah S, Kemp TJ, Erwteman A, et al. Outcome following open reduction and internal fixation of open pilon fractures. J Bone Joint Surg Am 2010; 92(2):346–52.
10. Chen SH, Wu PH, Lee YS. Long-term results of pilon fractures. Arch Orthop Trauma Surg 2007;127(1):55–60.
11. Watson JT, Moed BR, Karges DE, et al. Pilon fractures. Treatment protocol based on severity of soft tissue injury. Clin Orthop Relat Res 2000;(375):78–90.
12. Kilian O, Bundner MS, Horas U, et al. Long-term results in the surgical treatment of pilon tibial fractures. A retrospective study. Chirurg 2002;73(1):65–72.
13. Rammelt S, Endres T, Grass R, et al. The role of external fixation in acute ankle trauma. Foot Ankle Clin 2004;9(3):455–74. vii-viii.
14. Bacon S, Smith WR, Morgan SJ, et al. A retrospective analysis of comminuted intra-articular fractures of the tibial plafond: open reduction and internal fixation versus external Ilizarov fixation. Injury 2008;39(2):196–202.
15. Papadokostakis G, Kontakis G, Giannoudis PV, et al. External fixation devices in the treatment of fractures of the tibial plafond: a systematic review of the literature. J Bone Joint Surg Br 2008;90(1):1–6.
16. Rammelt S, Marti RK, Raaymakers ELFB, et al. Joint-preserving reconstruction of malunited pilon fractures. FussSprungg 2012;10(1):62–72.
17. Zwipp H, Rammelt S, Endres T, et al. High union rates and function scores at midterm followup with ankle arthrodesis using a four screw technique. Clin Orthop Relat Res 2010;468(4):958–68.
18. Rammelt S, Marti RK, Zwipp H. Joint-preserving osteotomy of malunited ankle and pilon fractures. Unfallchirurg 2013;116(9):789–96.

19. Ketz J, Sanders R. Staged posterior tibial plating for the treatment of Orthopaedic Trauma Association 43C2 and 43C3 tibial pilon fractures. J Orthop Trauma 2012; 26(6):341–7.
20. Liporace FA, Yoon RS. Decisions and staging leading to definitive open management of pilon fractures: where have we come from and where are we now? J Orthop Trauma 2012;26(8):488–98.
21. Bartoníček J, Mittlmeier T, Rammelt S. Anatomy, biomechanics and pathomechanics of the tibial pilon. FussSprungg 2012;10:3–11.
22. Weber M. Trimalleolar fractures with impaction of the posteromedial tibial plafond: implications for talar stability. Foot Ankle Int 2004;25(10):716–27.
23. Klammer G, Kadakia AR, Joos DA, et al. Posterior pilon fractures: a retrospective case series and proposed classification system. Foot Ankle Int 2013;34(2): 189–99.
24. Bartoníček J, Rammelt S, Kostlivy K, et al. Anatomy and classification of the posterior tibial fragment in ankle fractures. Arch Orthop Trauma Surg 2015;135(4): 505–16.
25. Weller S, Knapp U, Eck T. Ergebnisse nach Korrektureingriffen am oberen Sprunggelenk. Unfallheilkunde 1977;80:213–21.
26. Weise K, Weller S. Supramalleoläre Korrekturosteotomien. In: Strecker W, Keppler P, Kinzl L, editors. Posttraumatische Beindeformitäten. Analyse und Korrektur. Berlin; Heidelberg (Germany); New York: Springer; 1997. p. 215.
27. Rosen H. (Late) Reconstructive procedures about the ankle joint. In: Jahss MH, editor. Disorders of the foot and ankle, vol. III, 2nd edition. Philadelphia: Saunders; 1991. p. 2593–613.
28. Zwipp H. Chirurgie des Fußes. Wien (Austria); New York: Springer; 1994.
29. Marti RK. Correction of malunited ankle fractures. In: Marti RK, Heerwaarden RV, editors. Osteotomies for posttraumatic deformities. Stuttgart (Germany); New York: Thieme; 2008. p. 617–49.

Osteotomies of the Talar Neck for Posttraumatic Malalignment

Alexej Barg, MD[a],*, Thomas Suter, MD[b], Florian Nickisch, MD[a],
Nicholas J. Wegner, MD[a], Beat Hintermann, MD[b],*

KEYWORDS

- Talus fracture • Talar neck fracture • Hawkins classification
- Talar neck malalignment • Talar neck osteotomy

KEY POINTS

- A talar neck malunion is one of the major complications following operative or nonoperative treatment of talar neck fractures.
- The most common posttraumatic talar malunion results in varus malalignment of the talar neck and can lead to painful overload of the lateral foot and substantial impairment of hindfoot function.
- Secondary procedures in patients with painful malunited talar neck fracture include salvage procedures and anatomic reconstruction procedures.
- Anatomic reconstruction of the talar neck is a reliable surgical treatment to regain function, decrease pain, and restore hindfoot alignment and range of motion.

INTRODUCTION

Talus fractures are rare injuries and compose less than 1% of all fractures.[1,2] Talar neck fractures make up 50% of all talus injuries,[2,3] often caused by decelerating forces in combination with axial impaction.[4,5] In the current literature, there are numerous classification systems to describe talus fractures.[2] The most commonly cited classification is the Hawkins classification (**Fig. 1**), which was proposed in 1970 based on the degree of fracture displacement and dislocation of the tibiotalar and subtalar joints.[6] The initial Hawkins classification differentiated 3 types of talar neck fractures[6]: type I, nondisplaced fracture; type II, a talar neck fracture associated with a dislocation of the subtalar joint; and type III, a talar neck fracture and

The authors have nothing to disclose.
[a] Department of Orthopaedics, University of Utah, 590 Wakara Way, Salt Lake City, UT 84108, USA; [b] Department of Orthopaedics and Trauma, Kantonsspital Baselland, Rheinstrasse 26, Liestal CH-4410, Switzerland
* Corresponding authors.
E-mail addresses: alexej.barg@hsc.utah.edu; beat.hintermann@ksbl.ch

http://dx.doi.org/10.1016/j.fcl.2015.09.010
1083-7515/16/$ – see front matter © 2016 Elsevier Inc. All rights reserved.
foot.theclinics.com

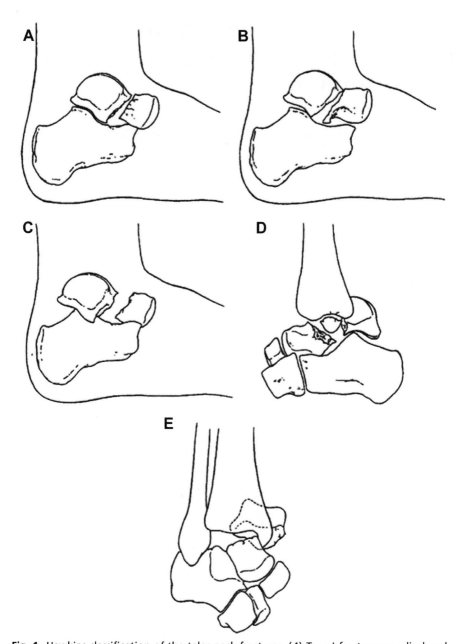

Fig. 1. Hawkins classification of the talar neck fractures. (*A*) Type I fracture: nondisplaced; (*B*, *C*) type II fracture: dislocation at the subtalar joint; (*D*) type III fracture: dislocation at the subtalar and tibiotalar joints; (*E*) type IV fracture: dislocation at the subtalar, tibiotalar, and talonavicular joints. (*From* Juliano PJ, Dabbah M, Harris TG. Talar neck fractures. Foot Ankle Clin 2004;9(4):727; with permission.)

dislocation at the subtalar and tibiotalar joints. In 1978, Canale and Kelly[7] modified the Hawkins classification by adding a type IV fracture: dislocation of the subtalar, tibiotalar, and talonavicular joints. Numerous clinical studies have demonstrated good reproducibility of the classification system and high prognostic value of Hawkins classification in terms of the clinical outcome and the occurrence of avascular necrosis of the talus.[8–13]

POSTTRAUMATIC TALAR NECK MALALIGNMENT

The reported rates of the posttraumatic malunion following talus fracture range from 0% to 67% (**Table 1**), with the most common posttraumatic talar malunion resulting in varus malalignment of the talar neck.[1–3,14–17] This varus malalignment often results in substantial shortening of the medial column with impairment of hindfoot motion as the hindfoot is locked in varus and internal rotation.[14,18,19] Sangeorzan and colleagues[20] performed a cadaveric study to evaluate the correlation between the degree of varus malalignment of the talar neck and the changes in contact characteristics of the subtalar joint. They demonstrated that the talar neck malalignment of as little as 2 mm results in substantial load redistribution between the posterior, middle, and anterior facets of the subtalar joint.[20] Daniels and colleagues[14] using a cadaveric model created an average varus malalignment of $17.1° \pm 2.4°$. This change in alignment led to a decrease of the average range of motion of the subtalar joint from $17.5° \pm 2.9°$ to $11.9° \pm 2.4°$.

Clinical studies have demonstrated that patients with talar malunions have poor outcomes related to overload of the lateral foot with painful callus formation on the lateral plantar side.[16,35] Patients present with substantially reduced range of motion in the subtalar and midtarsal joints often resulting in a painful, rigid foot with a cavovarus alignment. The talar neck malalignment may increase the chance of posttraumatic osteoarthritis in the peritalar joint. This condition, in turn, may result in substantial disability in daily activities.[16,19]

INDICATIONS/CONTRAINDICATIONS

Malunited talar neck fractures resulting in shortening of the medial column with concomitant hindfoot varus and forefoot varus and adductus resulting in lateral column overload are the typical surgical indications for the realigning corrective osteotomy of the talar neck.

Absolute contraindications for this procedure include acute or chronic infections, skin lesion (eg, ulcers on the foot), avascular necrosis of the talus, and neuroarthropathy (eg, Charcot arthropathy of the midfoot or hindfoot). Relative contraindications for talar neck realignment osteotomies include osteoporosis, immunosuppressive therapy, and tobacco use.

PREOPERATIVE PLANNING
Clinical Examination

All previous medical reports including surgery notes, if available, are collected and analyzed, for example, with regard to the previous surgeries and surgical approaches. Patients' history is assessed including the following aspects: pain, limitations with daily activities, and limitation with sports and recreational activities.

The physical examination starts with careful inspection of the foot and ankle while walking and standing. Hindfoot stability is assessed manually with patients sitting using the anterior drawer test.[36] Ankle and hindfoot alignment is assessed with patients

Table 1
Literature review addressing malunion rate in patients with talar fractures

Study	Study Type	Number of Patients		Talar Fracture Treatment	Follow-up (y)[a]	Malunion Rate
		All Talar Fractures	Talar Neck Fractures[b]			
Abdelgaid & Ezzat[21] 2012	RS, SC	16	16: type II, 10; type III, 4; type IV, 2	16 percutaneous reduction and 3.5-mm cannulated screw fixation	4.0 (3–5)	1 of 16 (6.3%)
Abdelkafy et al[22] 2015	RS, SC	8	8: type II, 6; type III, 2	8 ORIF lag screw fixation	3.9 (2–7)	0 of 8 (0.0%)
Canale & Kelly[7] 1978	RS, SC	71	71: type I, 15; type II, 30; type III, 23; type IV, 3	42 closed/open reduction, 29 ORIF	12.7 (3–37)	18 of 71 (25.4%)
Comfort et al[23] 1985	RS, SC	36	36: type I, 14; type II, 14; type III, 5; type IV, 3	8 closed reduction, 28 ORIF	nr	0 of 0 (0.0%)
Dumont et al[24] 2007	RS, SC	41	41: type I, 6; type II, 17; type III, 7; type IV, 3; dislocated peripheral fractures, 8	39 ORIF screw fixation, 2 ORIF K wire fixation, 12 with additional external fixation	4.0 (1–6)	6 of 41 (14.6%)
Dunn et al[25] 1966	RS, SC	23	23	15 closed reduction, 8 ORIF	nr	5 of 23 (21.7%)
Fleuriau Chateau et al[26] 2002	RS, SC	23	23: type II, 10; type III, 12; type IV, 1	23 ORIF one or two 2.0- or 2.4-mm plates with additional 2.0-, 2.7-, or 3.5-mm lag screws	1.7 (0.5–4.3)	2 of 23 (8.7%) (mild extension, no varus malalignment)
Fournier et al[27] 2012	RS, MC	114	114: type I, 33; type II, 48; type III, 29; type IV, 4	nr	9.3 (0.6–29.3)	37 of 117 (32.5%)
Frawley et al[28] 1995	RS, SC	26	26	6 plaster immobilization alone, 6 manipulation and plaster, 10 ORIF K wire fixation, 6 ORIF screw fixation (with or without supplementary K wires)	(1–8)	3 of 26 (11.5%)

Study	Design	N	Hawkins classification	Treatment	FU (y)	AVN
Gonzalez et al,[29] 2011	RS, SC	3	3: type III, 3	3 ORIF screw and plate fixation	4.0	0 of 3 (0.0%)
Lindvall et al,[30] 2004	RS, SC	26	18: type II, 11; type III, 6; type IV, 1	26 ORIF with different fixation devices	6.1 (4.0–9.4)	5 of 26 (19.2%)
Lorentzen et al,[31] 1977	RS, SC	123	123: type I, 54; type II, 53; type III, 16	106 closed reduction, 15 ORIF, 1 subtalar arthrodesis, 1 partial excision	1.8 (0.6–6.1)	18 of 123 (14.6%)
Ohl et al,[15] 2011	RS, SC	20	10: type II, 3; type III, 5; type IV, 2	8 ORIF K wire fixation, 7 ORIF 3.5-mm or small Herbert fixation, 5 ORIF combination K wires/ screws	7.5 (min FU 2 y)	6 of 9 (66.7%) patients with talar neck Fx; 2 of 8 (25%) patients with talar body Fx (all 8 patients with varus malalignment)
Peterson et al,[4] 1977	RS, SC	46	46: type I, 13; type II, 22; type III, 11	31 closed reduction, 15 ORIF	6.0 (1.3–13.3)	13 of 46 (28.3%)
Sanders et al,[32] 2004	RS, SC	70	70: type II, 29; type III, 25; type IV, 16.	66 ORIF screw fixation, 4 talectomy	5.2 (2.0–10.5)	21 of 66 (31.8%)
Schulze et al,[33] 2002	RS, SC	80	46: type I, 10; type II, 18; type III, 17; type IV, 1	67 ORIF screw fixation, 4 ORIF K wire fixation, 2 primary arthrodesis, 6 fragment excision	6.0 (1–15)	1 of 46 (2.2%)
Vallier et al,[34] 2014	RS, SC	81	81: type I, 2; type II, 44; type III, 32; type IV, 3	79 ORIF small-fragment and mini-fragment implants	2.5 (0.9–10.0)	2 of 81 (2.5%)
Xue et al,[17] 2014	RS, SC	28	28: type II, 19; type III, 9	28 ORIF plate fixation	2.1 (1.5–4.2)	0 of 28 (0.0%)

Abbreviations: FU, follow-up; FX, fracture; K wire, Kirschner wire; MC, multicenter; min, minimum; nr, not reported; ORIF, open reduction internal fixation; RS, retrospective; SC, single center.
a Values are presented as mean with range.
b If available with Hawkins classification.[6]

standing. Ankle range of motion is determined with a goniometer placed along the lateral border of the leg and foot in the weight-bearing position.[37] The range of motion of the subtalar joint can be measured clinically using a goniometer placed posteriorly on the hindfoot.[38] However, the clinically measured subtalar range of motion should be interpreted critically, as it is often overestimated compared with the radiographic measurements.[39]

Radiographic Evaluation

The standard radiographic evaluation includes 4 weight-bearing radiographs: anteroposterior and lateral views of the ankle, mortise view of the ankle, and the Saltzman hindfoot alignment view (**Fig. 2**).[40] Only weight-bearing radiographs should be used for radiographic evaluation, as non–weight-bearing measurements are often misleading and not reliable.[41–43] The talonavicular alignment should be assessed by measurement of the talar–first metatarsal angle in the horizontal plane as described previously.[44] The anteroposterior talar–first metatarsal angle is considered negative if the first metatarsal is aligned in an adducted position with respect to the axis of the talus.

In 1978, Canale and Kelly[7] described a novel radiographic technique to evaluate the varus displacement and rotation of the talar head and neck. Using the Canale view, the talar neck is viewed in the frontal plane while the ankle is placed in maximum equinus with the foot in 15° pronation and the x-ray is angled 15° cephalad and centered on the talar neck.[7,45] The radiographic malalignment assessment using the Canale view should be interpreted carefully as the measured talar neck displacement and rotation is often underestimated.[46] The most accurate imaging technique to measure the talar neck malalignment has been shown to be computed tomography.[2,46] Furthermore, the comparison with the contralateral uninjured side can be helpful.

To assess the viability of the talus, the authors recommend using MRI.[47,48] In 1970, Hawkins[6] described radiolucency in the subchondral area of the talus between the sixth and eighth week following the injury, which indicates viability of the talar body, now called the Hawkins sign. Chen and colleagues[48] evaluated the prognostic value of the Hawkins sign in 44 patients with talar neck fracture. In this study, the Hawkins sign was shown as a reliable predictor excluding avascular necrosis of the talus.[48]

Single-photon emission computed tomography can be used for better assessment of localization and biological activity of degenerative changes in the peritalar joints.[49] Computed tomography can be helpful to assess the integrity and contour of bone, for preoperative planning of the corrective osteotomy.[19]

SURGICAL TECHNIQUE
Anesthesia and Patient Positioning

Realignment of the talar neck can be performed using general or regional anesthesia. Patients are placed supine with a bump under the ipsilateral hip until the foot is pointing perpendicular to the operating table. The iliac crest is draped free to allow harvesting of the autologous bone graft if necessary. A pneumatic tourniquet is applied on the ipsilateral thigh, and preoperative antibiotic prophylaxis is administered before inflation of the tourniquet.

Surgical Procedure

A dorsomedial approach is used to expose the malunited talar neck centered between the anterior and posterior tibial tendons or just medial to the anterior tibial tendon. In patients with previous surgeries, a modified approach through the prior

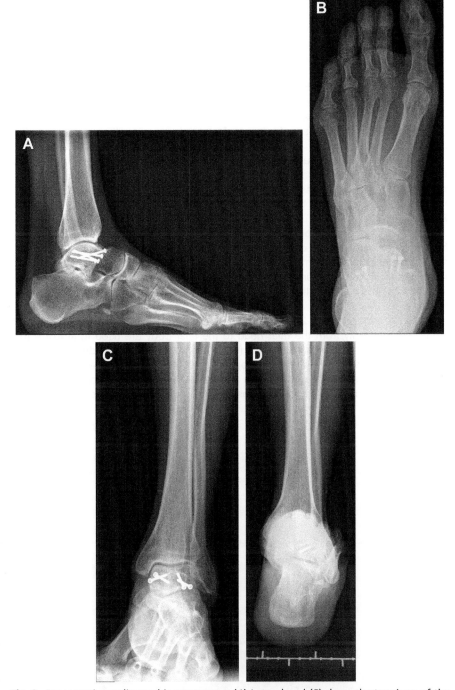

Fig. 2. Preoperative radiographic assessment. (*A*) Lateral and (*B*) dorsoplantar views of the foot. (*C*) Mortise view of the ankle. (*D*) Saltzman hindfoot alignment view radiographs show the left foot of a 51-year-old male patient with a malunited talar neck fracture. Open reduction and internal fixation of a Hawkins type II talar neck fracture was performed 2 years ago. Note the shortening of the medial column with supination/adduction deformity of the forefoot and hindfoot varus malalignment.

incision should be used, when the minimal distance between the old scar and the intended dorsomedial approach is less than 4 cm. In patients with previous talar neck osteosynthesis, all implants should be removed before performing the osteotomy.

The previous fracture plane is marked using Kirschner wires (K wires), and a chisel is used to complete the osteotomy along the fracture plane. In patients with contractures of the flexor digitorum longus tendon and posterior tibial tendon, a posteromedial release should be performed before lengthening the medial column.

Two K wires are then placed on both sides of the talar neck osteotomy, and a distractor is mounted over these two K wires. The authors use a Hintermann distractor (Integra LifeSciences Corporation, Plainsboro, NJ, USA), which allows not only controlled distraction but also rotational control of the talar neck and body (**Fig. 3**).

Once the underlying deformity of the talar neck is completely corrected through the medial opening wedge osteotomy, the resulting gap is measured using a ruler. In most cases, the gap is measured between 4 and 10 mm. The graft is then prepared based on the measured osteotomy gap. Either tricortical autograft from the iliac crest or a cancellous allograft block can be used for interposition at the osteotomy site.

As a standard approach, 2 position screws (3.5 mm, cannulated or solid) inserted distally to proximally from the talar head to the talar body are used to stabilize the inserted graft and talar neck osteotomy (**Fig. 4**). In some cases, an additional medial buttress plate is used, for example, if the bone graft may not provide enough distraction stability against compressive forces across the talar neck osteotomy. In patients with more distal fractures requiring an osteotomy close to the head of the talus, the

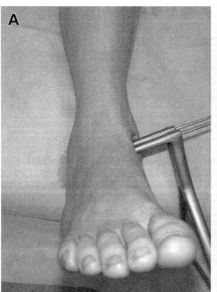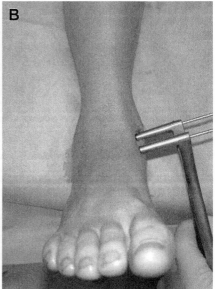

Fig. 3. Talar neck deformity correction using a special distractor. (A) Supination/adduction deformity of the forefoot in a 37-year-old female patient with a malunited talar neck fracture. (B) A special distractor is used to open the talar neck osteotomy resulting in complete correction of the underlying forefoot deformity.

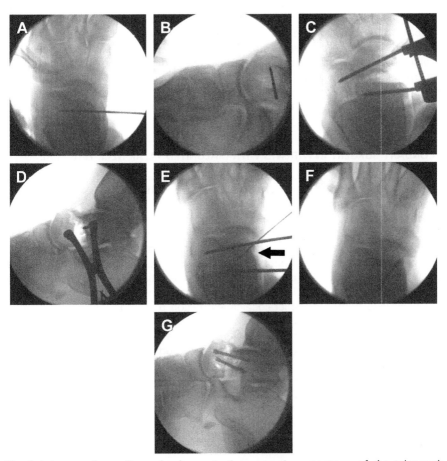

Fig. 4. Intraoperative radiographs demonstrating corrective osteotomy of the talar neck (the same patient from **Fig. 2**). (*A, B*) The osteotomy plane is marked using a K wire across the previous talar neck fracture. (*C, D*) A special distractor is applied over 2 K wires to perform distractional and rotational correction of the talar neck. (*E*) Dorsoplantar radiograph shows the inserted cancellous allograft block (*arrow*), which is fixed preliminarily using a K wire. (*F, G*) Dorsoplantar and lateral radiographs show the final fixation of the inserted allograft with two 3.5-mm cannulated screws.

distal fragment is often very short. In these cases, screw fixation may not provide enough stability against rotational forces because of the limited size of the distal osteotomy fragment. In those cases, the combined fixation using an addition plate or staples can be performed.

In patients with concomitant osteoarthritis of the adjacent joints, arthrodesis or debridement of the subtalar and/or talonavicular joints should be performed. If necessary, percutaneous lengthening of the Achilles tendon should be performed to achieve physiologic ankle range of motion. Finally, wound closure is performed sequentially.

Aftercare

After surgery, a well-padded short leg splint is used to hold the operated foot/ankle in the neutral position. When the wound is completely dry, typically 3 to 4 days after the surgery, patients are transitioned to a walking boot or to a short leg cast. Patients are restricted to partial weight bearing for a total of 8 weeks following surgery. Then, an intensive rehabilitation program is started after walker or cast removal and continued for at least 4 months, including gait training, stretching and strengthening exercises, and local antiphlogistic measures, including lymphatic drainage. The authors recommend thromboembolism prophylaxis using subcutaneous application of low-molecular-weight heparin until patients are fully weight bearing without a cast or walking boot.

SECONDARY SURGERY IN PATIENTS WITH MALUNITED TALAR NECK FRACTURE
Salvage Procedures

Numerous salvage procedures have been described in the current literature for malunited talar neck fractures, including peritalar arthrodesis (ankle arthrodesis, subtalar and/or talonavicular arthrodesis, triple arthrodesis), total ankle replacement (patients with ankle osteoarthritis resulting from the injury or associated avascular necrosis), and tibiocalcaneal arthrodesis with or without talectomy (**Table 2**).[1,7,10,13,16,17,28,32,50–55]

Canale and Kelly[7] treated 4 patients with painful varus talar neck malunion with a triple arthrodesis at 3, 6, 24, and 28 months after the initial surgery. The final results were reported as good in all 4 cases. Another patient with varus malunion of the talar neck was treated by tibiotalocalcaneal fusion 5 months following the initial injury resulting in a good outcome at the final follow-up.[7] Frawley and colleagues[28] reported the midterm outcome between 1 and 8 years postoperatively in 26 patients with talar fractures. In total, secondary procedures were required in 7 patients, most commonly in patients with substantial displacement of fracture fragments. These secondary procedures included 3 subtalar arthrodeses, 3 triple arthrodeses, and 1 ankle arthrodesis.[28] Kitaoka and Patzer[54] performed an ankle arthrodesis in 19 patients with posttraumatic ankle arthritis and talus osteonecrosis following talus fracture. At the mean follow-up of 6 years, the clinical results were excellent in 7 patients, good in 6, fair in 3, and poor in 3 patients. Union occurred

Table 2
Literature review addressing outcome of secondary salvage procedures in patients with talar neck malalignment

Study	Study Type	Patients with Talar Neck Malalignment	Secondary Surgery	Outcome
Asencio et al,[50] 2000	RS, SC	11	Peritalar AD (11)	Reported as good in all 11 cases
Canale & Kelly,[7] 1978	RS, SC	5	Triple AD (4), TTC AD (1)	Reported as good in all 5 cases
Frawley et al,[28] 1995	RS, SC	7	Subtalar AD (3), triple AD (3), ankle AD (1)	Excellent (2), good (1), fair (2), poor (2)
Ohl et al,[15] 2011	RS, SC	1	Neck OT and subtalar AD (1)	AOFAS score 59
Sanders et al,[32] 2004	RS, SC	5	Triple AD (3), subtalar AD (2)	nr
Xue et al,[17] 2014	RS, SC	5	Subtalar AD (3), ankle AD (1), TAR (1)	nr

Abbreviations: AD, arthrodesis; AOFAS, American Orthopaedic Foot and Ankle Society; nr, not reported; OT, osteotomy; RS, retrospective; SC, single center; TAR, total ankle replacement; TTC, tibiotalocalcaneal.

in 16 of the 19 ankles.[54] Rockett and colleagues[55] presented a case report of a talar neck nonunion following a Hawkins type II talar neck fracture treated with a triple arthrodesis with good postoperative results at 1 year. Asencio and colleagues[50] treated 11 patients with nonunion or malunion following talar neck fracture with peritalar arthrodesis. In most cases, complete bone healing and deformity correction was observed.[50] Sanders and colleagues[32] reported the outcome in 17 patients treated by open reduction and screw fixation for displaced talar neck fractures. In 5 patients malunion with concomitant degenerative changes occurred, which has been treated by triple or subtalar arthrodesis in 3 and 2 patients, respectively.[32] Xue and colleagues[17] treated 31 patients with displaced talar neck fractures using plate fixation through dual approaches. Secondary surgeries were performed in 5 patients, including 3 subtalar arthrodeses, 1 ankle arthrodesis, and 1 total ankle replacement.[17] Ohl and colleagues[15] reported the long-term results after surgical treatment of talar fractures in 20 patients. One patient with an initial Hawkins type III fracture developed a varus malunion of the talar neck with concomitant subtalar osteoarthritis, which was treated with corrective osteotomy and subtalar arthrodesis.[15]

Secondary Anatomic Reconstruction

In the last 2 decades, the secondary anatomic reconstruction of the malunited talar neck has been described in patients with preserved joint cartilage and without evidence of talar collapse, substantial avascular talar necrosis, or infection (**Table 3**).[1,15,16,18,35,56–59]

Monroe and Manoli[35] published a case report in 1999 describing a talar neck osteotomy using a tricortical iliac crest bone graft in a 34-year old male patient with a varus malunion following Hawkins type II talar neck fracture. The surgical reconstruction was performed 8 months after the initial conservative treatment. At a final follow-up of 4.7 years, the patient was very satisfied with the result and the average American Orthopaedic Foot and Ankle Society (AOFAS) hindfoot score improved from 11 to 85 points.[35] Huang and Cheng[56] published their results in 9 patients treated for neglected or mal-reduced talar fractures. Six patients had talar neck fractures; 2 patients had combined talar neck and talar body fracture; and 1 patient had a fracture of the posteromedial process of the talus. Surgical treatment included open reduction with or without bone grafting in 6 cases, ankle arthrodesis in 1 case,

Table 3
Literature review addressing outcomes of secondary anatomic reconstruction procedures in patients with talar neck malalignment

Study	Study Type	Patients with Talar Neck Malalignment	Secondary Surgery	Outcome
Huang & Cheng,[56] 2005	RS, SC	6	ORIF & bone graft (3), ORIF (2), neck OT (1)	AOFAS score 77 ± 13 (54–97); AVN requiring ankle AD (1), delayed wound healing (1)
Rammelt et al,[60] 2005	PS, SC	7	Neck OT (7)	AOFAS score 86, Maryland Foot Score 87

Abbreviations: AD, arthrodesis; AOFAS, American Orthopaedic Foot and Ankle Society; AVN, avascular necrosis; ORIF, open reduction internal fixation; OT, osteotomy; PS, prospective; RS, retrospective; SC, single center.

Table 4	
Classification of posttraumatic talar deformities	
Type I	Malunion and/or Joint displacement
Type II	Nonunion with joint displacement
Type III	Types I/II with partial avascular necrosis
Type IV	Types I/II with complete avascular necrosis
Type V	Types I/II with septic avascular necrosis

Secondary anatomic reconstruction may be contemplated in compliant patients with type I/III deformities with good bone and cartilage quality.

Adapted from Rammelt S, Winkler J, Heineck J, et al. Anatomic reconstruction of malunited talus fractures: a prospective study of 10 patients followed for 4 years. Acta Orthop 2005;76(4):589; and Zwipp H, Rammelt S. Posttraumatic deformity correction at the foot. Zentralbl Chir 2003;128(3):221; [in German]; with permission.

talar neck osteotomy in 1 case, and a combination of talar neck osteotomy with subtalar arthrodesis in 1 case. In all cases, the fracture healed. At a mean follow-up of 4.4 years, the mean AOFAS hindfoot score was 77.4 points. One patient subsequently developed avascular necrosis of the talus.[56] Rammelt and colleagues[60] treated 10 patients with painful talar malunions following 7 talar neck fractures (3 Hawkins type II fractures, 3 Hawkins type III fractures, and 1 Hawkins type I fracture) and 3 talar body fractures. The investigators described a novel classification of posttraumatic talar deformities (**Table 4**). In patients with malunited talar neck fractures, an anteromedial approach was used and corrective osteotomy along the former fracture plane was performed. The autologous bone grafting from the ipsilateral iliac crest was used to fill the osteotomy gap. No postoperative complications were observed in the entire patient cohort. The mean AOFAS hindfoot score significantly increased from 38 points preoperatively to 86 points postoperatively. The mean

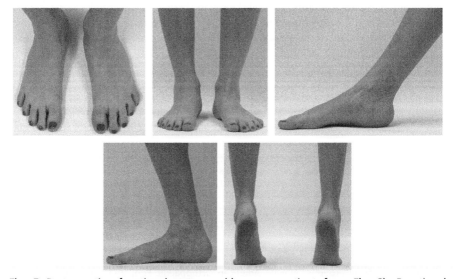

Fig. 5. Postoperative functional outcome (the same patient from **Fig. 3**). Functional outcome at the 2-year follow-up after reconstructive osteotomy of the talar neck.

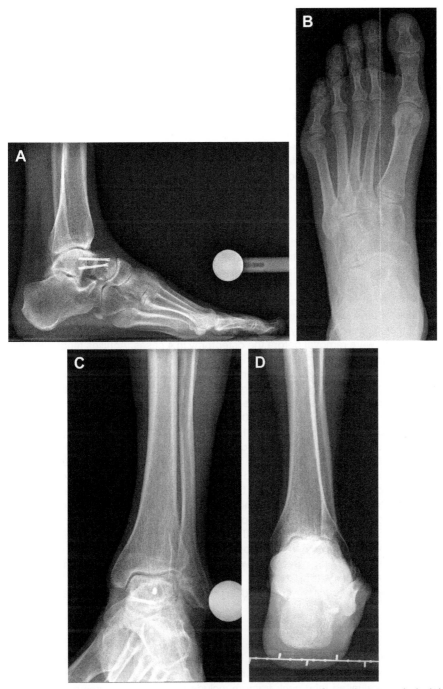

Fig. 6. Postoperative radiographic outcome (the same patient from **Figs. 2** and **4**). (*A*) Lateral and (*B*) dorsoplantar views of the foot, (*C*) mortise view of the ankle, and (*D*) Saltzman hindfoot alignment view radiograph at 3-year follow-up after reconstructive osteotomy of the talar neck. Note the complete osseous healing at the site of the osteotomy and physiologic alignment of foot/hindfoot in all 3 planes.

Maryland Foot Score significantly increased from 44 points preoperatively to 87 points postoperatively. There were no cases of postoperative avascular necrosis; in patients with preexisting partial avascular necrosis, no progression of the necrosis was detected. All but 1 patient was very satisfied with the obtained results.[60] Seven years later in 2012, Rammelt and Zwipp[57] updated their results in a series of 22 joint-preserving corrections in patients with posttraumatic talar malunions. Twenty of 22 patients were assessed clinically and radiographically at the mean follow-up of 4.8 years with a range between 1.5 and 14.0 years. The mean AOFAS hindfoot score significantly increased from 36.9 points preoperatively to 87.5 points postoperatively. In 12 of 20 patients, there was progression of peritalar arthritis. Three patients eventually required hindfoot fusion: 1 ankle arthrodesis, 1 talonavicular arthrodesis, and 1 two-stage ankle and subtalar arthrodesis at 7.5, 5.0, and 1.5 years, respectively.[57]

RESULTS

In 2013, the authors reported the midterm results in 7 patients with malunited talar neck fracture treated with a talar neck osteotomy to lengthen the medial column of the foot.[19] There were 5 male and 2 female patients with a mean age of 42 years with a range between 17 and 60 years. The initial treatment of the talar neck fracture was open reduction and internal fixation using K wires or screw fixation in 4 patients and nonoperative management in 3 patients. The corrective osteotomy was performed using the previously described surgical technique. Additional surgeries included hardware removal before the osteotomy in 4 cases, Achilles tendon lengthening in 2 cases, medial and/or posterior release in 2 cases, arthroscopy of the subtalar joint in 1 case, and subtalar arthrodesis in 1 case. The mean follow-up in this retrospective study was 4 years ranging between 2.5 and 9.8 years. All patients experienced significant pain relief with a decrease in their pain visual analog scale (VAS) from 7.4 ± 1.0 preoperatively to 1.7 ± 0.8 postoperatively. The mean range of motion of the tibiotalar joint increased from $41° \pm 9°$ preoperatively to $44° \pm 8°$ postoperatively, whereas the mean range of motion of the subtalar joint substantially decreased from $22° \pm 6°$ preoperatively to $17° \pm 7°$ postoperatively (**Fig. 5**). The mean AOFAS hindfoot score significantly increased from 40.9 ± 18.8 points preoperatively to 83.9 ± 11.1 points postoperatively. At the latest follow-up, all patients were satisfied with the postoperative outcomes and no avascular necrosis or progression of degenerative changes were observed in the patient cohort. The mean talar–first metatarsal angle in the horizontal plane significantly increase from $11.9° \pm 7.3°$ preoperatively to $0.9° \pm 4.7°$ postoperatively. In all but one patient, radiographic evidence of osseous healing at the talar neck osteotomy was observed within 2 to 3 months after the reconstructive surgery (**Fig. 6**). One patient developed a talar neck osteotomy nonunion and required a subtalar and talonavicular fusion with complete relief of symptoms.

SUMMARY

Treatment of posttraumatic malunions following talar neck fractures is a challenging problem for the orthopedic surgeon. The secondary procedures in patients with painful malunited talar neck fracture include salvage procedures and anatomic reconstruction of the talar neck. The anatomic reconstruction has the major advantage in restoring the normal foot function in patients with preserved cartilage in peritalar joints and without evidence of extensile talar necrosis, collapse, or infection. Major concerns regarding the corrective talar neck osteotomy include intraoperative complications, nonunion, and the development or progression of avascular necrosis of the talus or peritalar degenerative changes. To date, no intraoperative complications have been described; only low rates of postoperative nonunion and/or avascular necrosis and peritalar osteoarthritis have been reported.

Corrective talar neck osteotomy results in reliable and satisfying clinical and radiographic results in patients with malunited talar neck fractures. However, only a limited number of retrospective case series exists reporting the outcome of this procedure. All these level IV evidence studies have significant limitations, including a small number of patients and only having a short-term or midterm follow-up duration. Therefore, further prospective, long-term follow-up studies with a larger number of patients should be performed to confirm the findings of previous studies.

REFERENCES

1. Calvert E, Younger A, Penner M. Post talus neck fracture reconstruction. Foot Ankle Clin 2007;12(1):137–51.
2. Rammelt S, Zwipp H. Talar neck and body fractures. Injury 2009;40(2):120–35.
3. Juliano PJ, Dabbah M, Harris TG. Talar neck fractures. Foot Ankle Clin 2004;9(4): 723–36.
4. Peterson L, Goldie IF, Irstam L. Fracture of the neck of the talus. A clinical study. Acta Orthop Scand 1977;48(6):696–706.
5. Peterson L, Romanus B, Dahlberg E. Fracture of the collum tali–an experimental study. J Biomech 1976;9(4):277–9.
6. Hawkins LG. Fractures of the neck of the talus. J Bone Joint Surg Am 1970;52(5): 991–1002.
7. Canale ST, Kelly FB Jr. Fractures of the neck of the talus. Long-term evaluation of seventy-one cases. J Bone Joint Surg Am 1978;60(2):143–56.
8. Alton T, Patton DJ, Gee AO. Classifications in brief: the Hawkins classification for talus fractures. Clin Orthop Relat Res 2015;473(9):3046–9.
9. Drummond Filho ML, Verzani MA, Rosa AF, et al. Fractures of the neck of the talus: evaluation of reproducibility of Hawkins' classification. Acta Ortop Bras 2012;20(3):170–3.
10. Halvorson JJ, Winter SB, Teasdall RD, et al. Talar neck fractures: a systematic review of the literature. J Foot Ankle Surg 2013;52(1):56–61.
11. Inokuchi S, Ogawa K, Usami N, et al. Long-term follow up of talus fractures. Orthopedics 1996;19(5):477–81.
12. Tezval M, Dumont C, Sturmer KM. Prognostic reliability of the Hawkins sign in fractures of the talus. J Orthop Trauma 2007;21(8):538–43.
13. Vallier HA, Nork SE, Barei DP, et al. Talar neck fractures: results and outcomes. J Bone Joint Surg Am 2004;86-A(8):1616–24.
14. Daniels TR, Smith JW, Ross TI. Varus malalignment of the talar neck. Its effect on the position of the foot and on subtalar motion. J Bone Joint Surg Am 1996; 78(10):1559–67.
15. Ohl X, Harisboure A, Hemery X, et al. Long-term follow-up after surgical treatment of talar fractures: twenty cases with an average follow-up of 7.5 years. Int Orthop 2011;35(1):93–9.
16. Sproule JA, Glazebrook MA, Younger AS. Varus hindfoot deformity after talar fracture. Foot Ankle Clin 2012;17(1):117–25.
17. Xue Y, Zhang H, Pei F, et al. Treatment of displaced talar neck fractures using delayed procedures of plate fixation through dual approaches. Int Orthop 2014; 38(1):149–54.

18. Rammelt S, Winkler J, Grass R, et al. Reconstruction after talar fractures. Foot Ankle Clin 2006;11(1):61–84.
19. Suter T, Barg A, Knupp M, et al. Surgical technique: talar neck osteotomy to lengthen the medial column after a malunited talar neck fracture. Clin Orthop Relat Res 2013;471(4):1356–64.
20. Sangeorzan BJ, Wagner UA, Harrington RM, et al. Contact characteristics of the subtalar joint: the effect of talar neck misalignment. J Orthop Res 1992;10(4):544–51.
21. Abdelgaid SM, Ezzat FF. Percutaneous reduction and screw fixation of fracture neck talus. Foot Ankle Surg 2012;18(4):219–28.
22. Abdelkafy A, Imam MA, Sokkar S, et al. Antegrade-retrograde opposing lag screws for internal fixation of simple displaced talar neck fractures. J Foot Ankle Surg 2015;54(1):23–8.
23. Comfort TH, Behrens F, Gaither DW, et al. Long-term results of displaced talar neck fractures. Clin Orthop Relat Res 1985;199:81–7.
24. Dumont C, Fuchs M, Burchhardt H, et al. What are the clinical results of operated fractures of the talus? Z Orthop Unfall 2007;145(2):212–20 [in German].
25. Dunn AR, Jacobs B, Campbell RD Jr. Fractures of the talus. J Trauma 1966;6(4):443–68.
26. Fleuriau Chateau PB, Brokaw DS, Jelen BA, et al. Plate fixation of talar neck fractures: preliminary review of a new technique in twenty-three patients. J Orthop Trauma 2002;16(4):213–9.
27. Fournier A, Barba N, Steiger V, et al. Total talar fracture - long-term results of internal fixation of talar fractures. A multicentric study of 114 cases. Orthop Traumatol Surg Res 2012;98(4 Suppl):S48–55.
28. Frawley PA, Hart JA, Young DA. Treatment outcome of major fractures of the talus. Foot Ankle Int 1995;16(6):339–45.
29. Gonzalez A, Stern R, Assal M. Reduction of irreducible Hawkins III talar neck fracture by means of a medial malleolar osteotomy: a report of three cases with a 4-year mean follow-up. J Orthop Trauma 2011;25(5):e47–50.
30. Lindvall E, Haidukewych G, Dipasquale T, et al. Open reduction and stable fixation of isolated, displaced talar neck and body fractures. J Bone Joint Surg Am 2004;86-A(10):2229–34.
31. Lorentzen JE, Christensen SB, Krogsoe O, et al. Fractures of the neck of the talus. Acta Orthop Scand 1977;48(1):115–20.
32. Sanders DW, Busam M, Hattwick E, et al. Functional outcomes following displaced talar neck fractures. J Orthop Trauma 2004;18(5):265–70.
33. Schulze W, Richter J, Russe O, et al. Surgical treatment of talus fractures: a retrospective study of 80 cases followed for 1-15 years. Acta Orthop Scand 2002;73(3):344–51.
34. Vallier HA, Reichard SG, Boyd AJ, et al. A new look at the Hawkins classification for talar neck fractures: which features of injury and treatment are predictive of osteonecrosis? J Bone Joint Surg Am 2014;96(3):192–7.
35. Monroe MT, Manoli A 2nd. Osteotomy for malunion of a talar neck fracture: a case report. Foot Ankle Int 1999;20(3):192–5.
36. Phisitkul P, Chaichankul C, Sripongsai R, et al. Accuracy of anterolateral drawer test in lateral ankle instability: a cadaveric study. Foot Ankle Int 2009;30(7):690–5.
37. Lindsjo U, Danckwardt-Lilliestrom G, Sahlstedt B. Measurement of the motion range in the loaded ankle. Clin Orthop Relat Res 1985;199:68–71.
38. Buckley RE, Hunt DV. Reliability of clinical measurement of subtalar joint movement. Foot Ankle Int 1997;18(4):229–32.

39. Pearce TJ, Buckley RE. Subtalar joint movement: clinical and computed tomography scan correlation. Foot Ankle Int 1999;20(7):428–32.

40. Saltzman CL, El-Khoury GY. The hindfoot alignment view. Foot Ankle Int 1995; 16(9):572–6.

41. Shereff MJ, Digiovanni L, Bejjani FJ, et al. A comparison of nonweight-bearing and weight-bearing radiographs of the foot. Foot Ankle 1990;10(6):306–11.

42. Tochigi Y, Suh JS, Amendola A, et al. Ankle alignment on lateral radiographs. Part 1: sensitivity of measures to perturbations of ankle positioning. Foot Ankle Int 2006;27(2):82–7.

43. Tochigi Y, Suh JS, Amendola A, et al. Ankle alignment on lateral radiographs. Part 2: reliability and validity of measures. Foot Ankle Int 2006;27(2):88–92.

44. Younger AS, Sawatzky B, Dryden P. Radiographic assessment of adult flatfoot. Foot Ankle Int 2005;26(10):820–5.

45. Linklater JM, Read JW, Hayter CL. Chapter 3 imaging of the foot and ankle. In: Coughlin MJ, Saltzman CL, Anderson RB, editors. Mann's surgery of the foot and ankle. 9th edition. Philadelphia: Elsevier Saunders; 2014. p. 61–120.

46. Chan G, Sanders DW, Yuan X, et al. Clinical accuracy of imaging techniques for talar neck malunion. J Orthop Trauma 2008;22(6):415–8.

47. Babu N, Schuberth JM. Partial avascular necrosis after talar neck fracture. Foot Ankle Int 2010;31(9):777–80.

48. Chen H, Liu W, Deng L, et al. The prognostic value of the Hawkins sign and diagnostic value of MRI after talar neck fractures. Foot Ankle Int 2014;35(12):1255–61.

49. Pagenstert GI, Barg A, Leumann AG, et al. SPECT-CT imaging in degenerative joint disease of the foot and ankle. J Bone Joint Surg Br 2009;91(9):1191–6.

50. Asencio G, Rebai M, Bertin R, et al. Pseudarthrosis and non-union of disjunctive talar fractures. Rev Chir Orthop Reparatrice Appar Mot 2000;86(2):173–80 [in French].

51. Bonnin MP, Laurent JR, Casillas M. Ankle function and sports activity after total ankle arthroplasty. Foot Ankle Int 2009;30(10):933–44.

52. Elgafy H, Ebraheim NA, Tile M, et al. Fractures of the talus: experience of two level 1 trauma centers. Foot Ankle Int 2000;21(12):1023–9.

53. Gagneux E, Gerard F, Garbuio P, et al. Treatment of complex fractures of the ankle and their sequelae using trans-plantar intramedullary nailing. Acta Orthop Belg 1997;63(4):294–304 [in French].

54. Kitaoka HB, Patzer GL. Arthrodesis for the treatment of arthrosis of the ankle and osteonecrosis of the talus. J Bone Joint Surg Am 1998;80(3):370–9.

55. Rockett MS, De Yoe B, Gentile SC, et al. Nonunion of a Hawkin's group II talar neck fracture without avascular necrosis. J Foot Ankle Surg 1998;37(2):156–61 [discussion: 174].

56. Huang PJ, Cheng YM. Delayed surgical treatment for neglected or mal-reduced talar fractures. Int Orthop 2005;29(5):326–9.

57. Rammelt S, Zwipp H. Secondary correction of talar fractures: asking for trouble? Foot Ankle Int 2012;33(4):359–62.

58. Rammelt S, Zwipp H. Corrective arthrodeses and osteotomies for post-traumatic hindfoot malalignment: indications, techniques, results. Int Orthop 2013;37(9): 1707–17.

59. Zwipp H, Gavlik M, Rammelt S. Secondary anatomical reconstruction of malunited central talus fractures. Unfallchirurg 2014;117(9):767–75 [in German].

60. Rammelt S, Winkler J, Heineck J, et al. Anatomical reconstruction of malunited talus fractures: a prospective study of 10 patients followed for 4 years. Acta Orthop 2005;76(4):588–96.

Secondary Reconstruction for Malunions and Nonunions of the Talar Body

Hans Zwipp, MD, PhD, Stefan Rammelt, MD, PhD*

KEYWORDS

- Talus • Fracture • Malunion • Nonunion • Correction • Osteotomy

KEY POINTS

- Talar body malunions and nonunions lead to axial deviation and incongruity of both the ankle and subtalar joints, resulting in severe restriction of foot function.
- Anatomic reconstruction with joint preservation is feasible in compliant patients with good bone and cartilage quality.
- Bilateral approaches with adequate exposure of the talus and its joints and meticulous osteotomy technique are prerequisites for a good outcome.
- The few available studies show virtually no progression or development of avascular necrosis but some progression of posttraumatic arthritis with rates similar to that of primary internal fixation.
- Malunions and nonunions of the lateral or posterior talar process are mostly treated with excision of the malunited or loose fragments.

INTRODUCTION

Talar body fractures are severe and potentially disabling injuries. They are by definition intra-articular, and therefore even minor malunions will likely lead to malfunction of one or more of the peritalar joints that are essential for foot function.[1–3] Talar body fractures and thus malunions may be divided into central and peripheral fractures.[4] Central fractures of the talar body are typically produced by high-energy forces, while peripheral fractures (talar process fractures) result from shearing forces such as during subtalar dislocations.[5,6] Malunions and nonunions of central talar fractures frequently result from inadequate reduction and fixation, or nonoperative treatment of displaced

The authors have nothing to disclose.
Foot & Ankle Section, University Center for Orthopaedics & Traumatology, University Hospital Carl Gustav Carus at the TU Dresden, Fetscherstrasse 74, Dresden 01307, Germany
* Corresponding author.
E-mail address: strammelt@hotmail.com

talar body fractures,[7] while peripheral fractures of the lateral or posterior process may be overlooked in the wake of subtalar dislocations or other injuries.[5,8–11] Mills and Horne[12] noted a 60% nonunion rate after lateral process fractures were treated nonoperatively.

Even minor step-offs of 2 mm in the talar body will produce significant load shifts within the affected joint, potentially leading to posttraumatic arthritis.[13] Any axial deviation of the talar body will inevitably lead to a 3-dimensional malposition of the hindfoot, severely affecting overall foot function. Malunions of the lateral talar process may rapidly lead to subtalar arthritis.[10,11] Nonunions of the lateral process have to be discriminated from a symptomatic accessory talus. Posterior process malunions potentially lead to damage in both the ankle and subtalar joints.[8] Nonunions of the posterior process have to be discriminated from a loosened os trigonum or a bipartite talus.

In addition to malposition and instability caused by malunion and nonunion, the impact during the initial injury that is needed to produce a talar body fracture will inevitably result in chondrocyte death, further contributing to the development of post-traumatic arthritis. The rates of post-traumatic arthritis after central talar fractures provided in the literature vary considerably from 16% to 100% and appear to increase over time but only a about one-third of patients with radiographic signs of arthritis eventually becoming clinically symptomatic with the need for a secondary arthrodesis.[4]

Avascular necrosis (AVN) of the talar body is a specific complication after talar fractures. Its occurrence depends on the degree of initial dislocation and the overall severity of the injury. Undisplaced talar body fractures (Marti type II) are associated with AVN in 5% to 44% of patients, while displaced talar body fractures (Marti types III and IV) carry an overall risk of about 50%.[4] Open talar neck and body fractures appear to have an increased risk of AVN, while the time of definite fixation does not have a measurable impact.[14,15] When performing MRI on all displaced talar neck and body fractures, some areas of reduced blood supply will be found in virtually all cases.[16] However, only total AVN of the talar body subsequently leading to collapse of the talar dome becomes clinically relevant.[4,15,17] With only partial AVN, the necrotic areas of the talar body are gradually replaced by creeping substitution.[18] Infections occur in between 3% and 8% of cases, almost exclusively after open talar fractures.[2,14,15,18]

INDICATIONS/CONTRAINDICATIONS

Consequently, the presence of post-traumatic arthritis and the extent of AVN will form the basis of decision making when planning reconstruction for talar body malunions and nonunions.[19] Other important factors for decision making are bone quality and patient compliance. **Table 1** contains an easy-to-use classification that may be used as a guideline for treatment.

Joint-preserving corrections are aimed at regaining a maximum of function while correcting the deformity and reducing pain. They might be considered in the absence of manifest arthritis and with no or only partial AVN of the talar body (Type I–III deformities) in selected cases of active, compliant patients. Contraindications are relevant comorbidities such as poorly controlled diabetes mellitus, Stage IIb peripheral vascular disease, or systemic immune deficiency.

SURGICAL TECHNIQUE
Preoperative Planning

Patients with talar malunions and nonunions have to be evaluated clinically with respect to pain, gross deformity, soft tissue conditions, callosities, neurovascular status, range of motion and stability in the ankle, subtalar, and talonavicular joints.

Table 1
Classification and proposed treatment algorithm for talar malunions

		Treatment Options	
Type	Features	Active, Reliable Patient, No Symptomatic Arthritis	Noncompliant Patient, Comorbidities, Arthritis
I	Malunion with joint displacement	Osteotomy, secondary reconstruction, and internal fixation with joint preservation	Corrective fusion of the affected joint(s)
II	Nonunion with displacement		
III	Types I/II with partial AVN		
IV	Types I/II with complete AVN	Necrectomy, (vascularized) bone grafting, corrective fusion	
V	Types I/II with septic AVN	Radical debridement(s), bone grafting, corrective fusion	

Modified from Rammelt S, Winkler J, Heineck J, et al. Anatomical reconstruction of malunited talus fractures: a prospective study of 10 patients followed for 4 years. Acta Orthop 2005;76(4):588–96; and Zwipp H, Rammelt S. Posttraumatic deformity correction at the foot. Zentralbl Chir 2003;128(3):218–26. [in German].

Important patient-related factors to be considered are activity level, professional demands, comorbidities (above all osteoporosis, diabetes, and any neurovascular deficits), substance abuse, and inability to comply with the postoperative protocol.

Radiographic assessment of the overall alignment and stability includes bilateral weight-bearing anteroposterior, dorsoplantar, and lateral radiographs of the foot and ankle, and a hindfoot alignment view (**Fig. 1**). Computed tomography (CT) scanning is mandatory for planning the correction. It reveals the exact 3-dimensional outline of the malunited fragments and joint incongruities, as well as the extent of arthritis and bony union. MRI is used to determine the presence and extent of AVN,

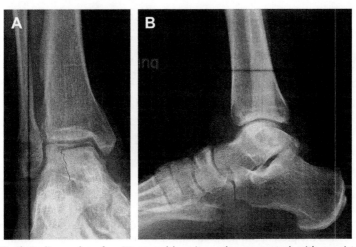

Fig. 1. (*A, B*) Radiographs of a 25-year-old waiter who presented with persistent pain 4 months after a fall from a staircase that was treated as an ankle sprain. The images show a step-off in the talar dome and some irregularity at the subtalar joint. (*Adapted from* Rammelt S, Zwipp H. Secondary correction of talar fractures: asking for trouble? Foot Ankle Int 2012;33(4):360; with permission.)

osteochondral defects, and associated soft-tissue pathologies like tendon impinge-ment (**Fig. 2**). Ongoing infection should be ruled out with routine leukocyte counts and C-reactive protein serum levels.

Because malalignment of the talar body and its joints will invariably cause pain around the ankle and hindfoot, it may be difficult to assess if radiologic evidence of post-traumatic arthritis is clinically relevant. Consequently, the decision to reconstruct or fuse one or more joints around the talus will frequently be made during reconstruc-tive surgery by visually assessing and directly probing the cartilage quality (**Fig. 3**). Both treatment options—fusion and joint reconstruction—must be discussed with the patient prior to surgery.

Malunions and nonunions of the lateral or posterior process can be salvaged at an early stage by complete excision of the malunited fragments and joint revision.[8,20] If severe arthritis of the subtalar joint is present already, in situ fusion is the treatment of choice.[11]

Surgical Approaches and Patient Positioning

Anatomic correction of malunited fractures of the talar body is generally carried out via the same surgical approaches that are used in acute fractures.[4,14,15] In analogy to acute talar body fractures, most malunions require bilateral approaches.[7,21] The medial and central aspect of the talar dome is visualized via an anteromedial approach and an additional medial malleolar osteotomy (see **Fig. 3**). An anterolateral approach is used to access the subtalar joint and lateral process. The patient is placed in a supine position with a bump placed beneath the ipsilateral hip to place the foot in a neutral

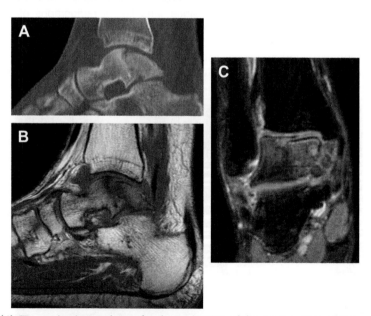

Fig. 2. (A) CT scanning is mandatory for determination of the exact outline of the malunion or nonunion and the presence of posttraumatic arthritis. In this case, a step-off in both the ankle and subtalar joints is obvious. Reconstruction will require bilateral approaches. (B, C) MRI shows edema of the talar body but no signs of extensive necrosis and still intact carti-lage at both joints (same patient as in **Fig. 1**). (*Adapted from* Rammelt S, Zwipp H. Secondary correction of talar fractures: asking for trouble? Foot Ankle Int 2012;33(4):361; with permission.)

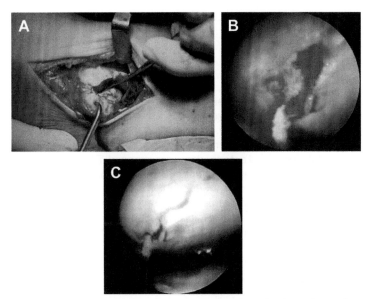

Fig. 3. (*A*) Intraoperative aspect of the large step-off in the talar dome but still intact cartilage cover as seen from the anteromedial approach after medial malleolar osteotomy. The talar body osteotomy is carried out step-wise with small chisels. (*B*, *C*) Anatomic reduction of the subtalar joint is controlled via an oblique lateral approach and additional dry arthroscopy. Minor incongruities can be corrected this way (same patient as in **Figs. 1–2**).

position. A posterolateral or posteromedial approach is needed in cases of malunions or nonunions of the posterior process and the posterior part of the talar body.[4,8] For these approaches, the patient is placed in a prone position. Proper use of the image intensifier must be assured (**Fig. 4**). In selected cases, intraoperative or postoperative

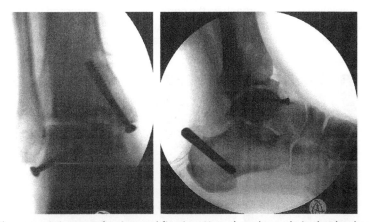

Fig. 4. Fluoroscopic images after internal fixation. Note the calcaneal pin that has been used for tibiocalcaneal distraction to improve exposition of the ankle and subtalar joints with the application of a femoral distractor. The medial malleolar osteotomy was fixed with 2 screws (same patient as in **Figs. 1–3**). (*Adapted from* Rammelt S, Zwipp H. Secondary correction of talar fractures: asking for trouble? Foot Ankle Int 2012;33(4):361; with permission.)

3-dimensional imaging is useful (**Fig. 5**) to verify anatomic reconstruction that will lead to a favorable outcome (**Fig. 6**).

SURGICAL PROCEDURES
Anterior and Central Talar Body

According to the preoperative analysis (**Fig. 7**), an anteromedial incision is carried out in a curved manner, starting approximately 3 cm above the medial malleolus and extending to the navicular tuberosity. The posterior tibial tendon is retracted inferiorly with a soft strap, and tenolysis is carried out, if necessary. The medial joint capsule is opened, and the talar neck and anterior dome are exposed. Fibrous adhesions around the talus are released. Most talar body fractures will need an additional medial malleolar osteotomy to reliably access and reduce the malunited fragments (**Fig. 8**). In the authors' preference, it is carried out as a Chevron osteotomy and obliquely running directly to the medial angle of the ankle joint. The holes for refixation of the medial malleolus with 2 screws are predrilled at that stage. The posterior tibial tendon is protected with a smooth retractor. The osteotomy is then carried out with an oscillating saw under direct vision of the medial aspect of the ankle joint. Care is taken not to dissect deltoid ligament behind the sustentaculum tali in order not to compromise the blood supply to the posterior talar body.[21]

Complete assessment of the talar body necessitates a second approach at its lateral aspect. The lateral approach can be carried out as a slightly curved anterolateral approach starting anterior to the distal fibula and running distally to the anterior calcaneal process just above the peroneal tendons. Alternatively, an oblique Ollier/Ducroquet approach is performed along the skin crests just anterior to the distal fibula over the sinus tarsi. Care is taken not to injure the lateral branch of the superficial peroneal nerve in the superior portion and the peroneal tendons in the inferior portion of the approach. The tendons are held away distally with a soft strap inside their sheath. Frequently there are adhesions and tendon impingement by displaced lateral process fragments and osteophytes that have to be released during corrective surgery. Visualization of the ankle and subtalar joints may be improved with the help of a spanning femoral distractor introduced between the distal tibia and the calcaneus.[1,7]

After completion of the approaches, the cartilage status is assessed by thorough inspection and probing of all accessible parts. Loose, nonviable fragments are excised. Smaller cartilaginous lesions may be treated with curettage and drilling or

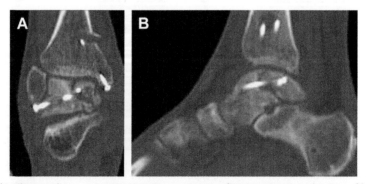

Fig. 5. (A, B) Immediate postoperative CT scanning confirms anatomic reduction of both the ankle and subtalar joints. The comminuted fragments at the medial aspect of the talar dome have not been addressed during surgery (same patient as in **Figs. 1–4**).

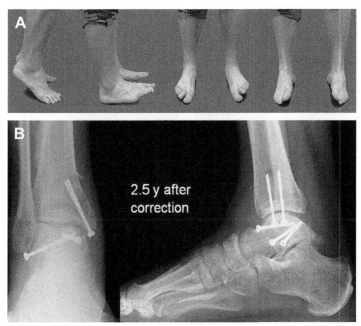

Fig. 6. (*A*) Two and a half years after corrective osteotomy, the patient has near-normal function of the ankle and subtalar joints. (*B*) Standing radiographs show bony union and no signs of post-traumatic arthritis (same patients as in **Figs. 1–5**). (*Adapted from* Rammelt S, Zwipp H. Secondary correction of talar fractures: asking for trouble? Foot Ankle Int 2012;33(4):361; with permission.)

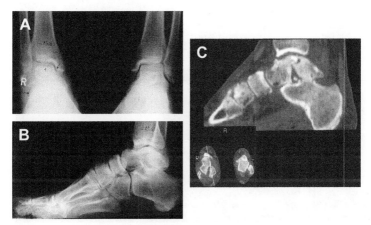

Fig. 7. A 42-year-old mechanic presents 3 months (13 weeks) with a neglected displaced talar body fracture after a fall from a height of 5 m. Standing radiographs show a double contour in the talar dome (*arrow* in *A*), a talar inclination with anterior impingement at the ankle, and irregularity at the subtalar joint (*B*). CT scanning reveals a large gap in the subtalar joint with small intercalary fragments and a displaced fracture exiting through the ankle joint (*C*).

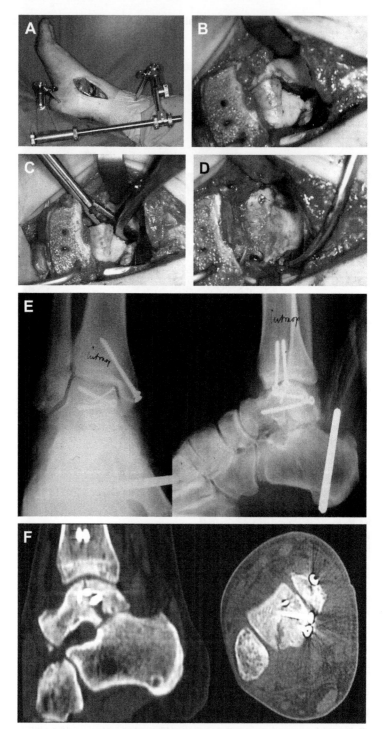

Fig. 8. (*A*) A medially placed femoral distractor between the tibia and the calcaneus is helpful in exposing the articular surfaces of the ankle and subtalar joints. (*B*) After completion of the medial approach, the gap and step-off in the ankle joint are seen (same patient as in **Fig. 7**). (*C*) The fracture has not united and is cleared from fibrous tissue, callus, and small intercalary fragments. (*D*) After anatomic correction, the fracture is fixed with screws. (*E, F*) Postoperative radiographs and CT scans demonstrate full restoration of ankle joint congruity while resection of the small intercalary fragments resulted in a gap in the subtalar joint.

microfracturing techniques. If a large, full-thickness defect is present at the weight-bearing area of the talus and/or adjacent bones, the decision to perform an arthrodesis of the affected joint(s) is made at this stage.

The malunited fracture sites are identified, and an osteotomy is carried out meticulously along the former fracture plane according to the preoperative planning with small osteotomes. The osteotomy is completed step-wise from medial and lateral under direct vision on the joint surface. Viability of the talar body may be checked at this stage with the tourniquet released. Smaller avascular areas of the talar body may be subjected to curettage and subchondral drilling to enhance bone regeneration.

Manifest nonunions of the talar body are treated with complete resection of the fibrous pseudarthrosis and curettage of the subchondral sclerotic bone until viable cancellous bone becomes visible. After reduction of the main fragments, the resulting defect is filled with cancellous bone graft from the distal tibia, the tibial head, or the iliac crest to avoid shortening or axial deviation.[11]

For anatomic reduction, the fragments are best manipulated with K-wires introduced from medial or lateral that may be used as joy sticks in order to avoid further damage to the joint surfaces or further fragmentation by direct manipulation with reduction clamps. Anatomic realignment of the talar body with reconstruction of the ankle and subtalar joints is checked visually through the bilateral approaches. The fragments are fixed temporarily with K-wires. Realignment of the talar body is controlled fluoroscopically. Parts of the subtalar joint that are not accessible with the bare eye despite distraction can be controlled with a small-diameter arthroscope.[22]

Definite fixation is achieved with small fragment (3.5 mm) or minifragment (2.0–2.7 mm) screws depending on the size of the fragments. If the former fracture extends largely into the talar neck or even head, leaving only a small anterior fragment, a minifragment plate is applied from 1 side, and screw fixation is employed on the other side. Alternatively, bilateral plates are used for better stabilization.[4]

Lateral Talar Process Malunions

Malunions and nonunions of the lateral talar process are accessed via a lateral oblique approach as detailed previously. Revision of the subtalar joint and resection of the malunited or pseudarthrotic fragment(s) (**Fig. 9**) serve as the treatment of choice.[11,20] The subtalar joint is cleared from loose or floating osteocartilagineous fragments. Focal cartilage defects may be subjected to curettage and microfracturing.

Posterior Talar Body and Posterior Talar Process

Depending on the exact fracture anatomy, a posterolateral or posteromedial approach is carried out for malunions and nonunions of the posterior talar body. As with acute fractures, placement of a tibiocalcaneal femoral distractor is most useful in order to obtain adequate overview over the posterior aspect of both the ankle and subtalar joints. The incision lies either lateral or medial to the Achilles tendon. Both approaches allow exposure of the whole posterior body of the talus. The choice is made based on the location and accessibility of the main posterior fragment and the planned direction of the screws. With the posterolateral approach, the sural nerve is identified in the proximal part of the incision, where it crosses from medial to lateral in the subcutaneous tissue. The superficial and deep fascia are incised, and the flexor hallucis longus muscle and tendon are carefully retracted medially, thus protecting the posterior neurovascular bundle that runs directly medial to it. Adhesions of the muscle, tendon, or posterior capsule are resected.

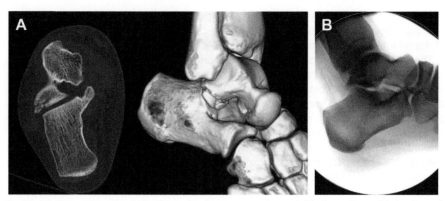

Fig. 9. (*A*) Nonunion of a lateral process fracture causing subfibular pain and irritation of the subtalar joint. (*B*) Complete resection of the loose or malunited fragments resulted in complete pain relief.

In analogy to the anterior talar body, the former fracture line is identified, and an osteotomy is carried out in case of a solid malunion, while a fibrous nonunion is resected. After anatomic reduction of both joint surfaces is confirmed, internal fixation is typically achieved with screws. Malunions or nonunions of the posterior talar process are treated with excision of the malunited or loose fragment(s).[11]

Immediate Postoperative Care

The operated foot is put in a splint or split below knee cast. Physical therapy with active and passive range of motion exercises starts early, usually on the second postoperative day, in order to maintain motion and prevent recurrence of adhesions. At 5 to 7 days, a walking cast, special boot, or walker is fitted, and patients are mobilized with partial weight bearing of about 20 kg, which roughly equals the weight of the leg when it is put to the ground but not loaded.

Rehabilitation and Recovery

After-treatment is tailored to the individual bone quality, the type of internal fixation, and the amount of bone grafting required during surgery. After osteotomy or bone grafting and internal fixation of the talar body, partial weight bearing with 20 kg is maintained for 10 to 12 weeks postoperatively in a lower leg cast or special arthrodesis boot.[1] Physical therapy is continued to achieve a near physiologic range of motion through the restored joints and a normal gait (**Fig. 10**). Removal of implants from the talus is usually not advised. Revision surgery may become necessary in case of restricted motion, protruding material, or progressive arthritis requiring fusion.[22]

Clinical Results in the Literature

Several authors report substantial improvement after resection of malunited fragments of the lateral process in the absence of manifest post-traumatic arthritis.[9,19,23] Veazey and colleagues[24] saw good-to-excellent results in 6 of 9 cases after resection of a nonunion of the posterior talar process. Two patients suffered from an affection of the sural nerve via the posterolateral approach, a complication that can be avoided by identifying and protecting the sural nerve in the subcutaneous tissue.

There are only few reports on the clinical results after secondary reconstruction for central talar body malunions and nonunions (**Table 2**). Most of the reported cases and

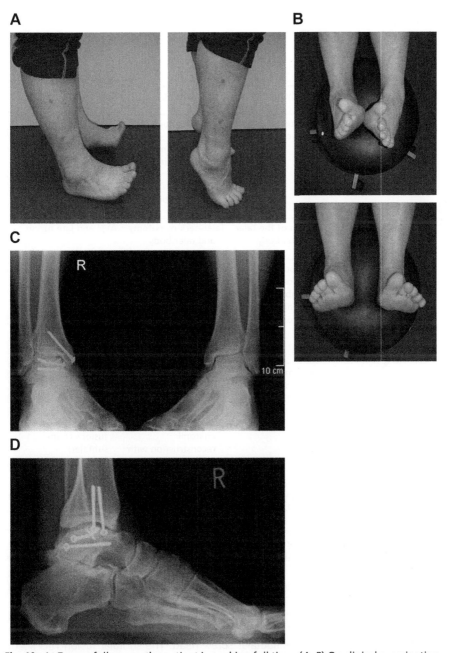

Fig. 10. At 7 years follow-up, the patient is working full time. (*A, B*) On clinical examination, the foot is well aligned, and the patient has almost normal ankle and subtalar range of motion. (*C, D*) The patient reports discomfort while walking on uneven ground and has some radiographic signs of subtalar arthritis but does not want any further surgery (same patient as in **Figs. 7** and **8**).

Table 2
Results after joint-preserving reconstruction for talar body malunion or nonunion. Corrective fusions were excluded

First Author, Year, Reference	n	Feature	Procedure	Reported Results
Asencio et al,[25] 2000	1	Talar body nonunion	Bone grafting	Bony union
Rammelt et al,[7] 2005	3	2 malunions, 1 nonunion	Osteotomy for malunion, debridement and bone grafting for nonunion, anatomic reconstruction with screws	No progression or development of AVN, good results at 4 y follow-up, 1 late ankle fusion (at 7.5 y)
Huang & Cheng,[26] 2005	1	Malunion of the talar neck and body	Talar neck osteotomy and talar body fixation	AVN and late fusion
Yu et al,[27] 2010	4	4 talar body malunions, (overall 13 combined talar body and neck malunion)	Osteotomy for malunion, debridement and bone grafting for nonunion, reduction and secondary screw fixaton	No progression or development of AVN, overall good results, 1 late fusion after combined talar neck and body malunion
Zwipp et al,[1] 2014[a]	9	6 malunions, 3 nonunions (5 Type I, 1 Type II, 3 Type III deformities)	Osteotomy for malunion, debridement and bone grafting for nonunion, anatomic reconstruction with screws/plates	No progression or development of AVN, average AOFAS score 87.6 at 6 y follow-up, 2 late fusions (1 ankle, 1 subtalar)

[a] Follow-up and continuation of the series can be found in Rammelt S, Winkler J, Heineck J, et al. Anatomical reconstruction of malunited talus fractures: a prospective study of 10 patients followed for 4 years. Acta Orthop 2005;76(4):588–96.

case series pertain to malunions of the talar neck, which are discussed in the article titled "Osteotomies of the talar neck for posttraumatic malalignment," by Barg and colleagues.[28] In 1992, Mahan and Lamy reported 1 case of a talar body nonunion with displacement.[24] The patient presented 9 months after the injury and closed reduction with a fixed equinus. Treatment consisted of open reduction via bilateral approaches, including medial malleolar osteotomy, internal fixation with screws, and subtalar fusion with additional bone grafting. At 18 months follow-up, he had mild pain at the ankle and around a subtalar screw head. The subtalar fusion was solid, but the talar fracture was still not completely united. Asencio and colleagues[25] described corrective surgery for 3 talar body malunions and nonunions. In 5 of 6 cases, correction was followed by fusion (2 subtalar fusions, 2 double fusions, and 1 triple fusion); in 1 case, a nonunion was treated successfully by bone grafting without fusion. On follow-up, 1 patient had a residual axial malalignment of 18°, and another patient had residual pain. Huang and Cheng[26] reported on 2 cases of combined talar neck and body malunions. One patient was treated with talar neck osteotomy and subtalar fusion, the other patient with talar neck osteotomy and secondary internal fixation of the talar body. The latter patient later developed AVN and ankle arthritis requiring ankle fusion. The authors concluded from their whole series, most cases being talar neck malunions, that delayed correction may lead to favorable results provided that no post-traumatic arthritis is present. This reflects the current authors' observations.[1,7,11] Yu and colleagues[27] reported on 24 patients with talar malunions and nonunions. Of these patients, 4 patients had initially suffered a talar body fracture, and 13 patients a combined talar neck and body fracture. The overall results were favorable, with only 1 patient needing a late subtalar fusion after correction of a combined talar body and neck malunion.

In 2005, the authors' group has provided a 4-year follow-up of the first 10 cases of anatomic reconstruction of talar malunions and nonunions, 3 of them at the talar body.[7] No development or progression of avascular necrosis was seen at that time point. More recently, an average 5-year follow-up of 23 cases of joint-sparing corrections after talar malunions and nonunions has been provided.[1] Of these patients, 9 patients had malunions and nonunions of the talar body. Two patients were female, and 7 patients were male, with a mean age of 35.6 years. Patients presented for correction at an average of 3 months after the injury. At an average of 6.1 years follow-up, the average AOFAS Ankle Hindfoot Scale was 87.6, as compared with 35.8 prior to correction. One patient needed an ankle fusion 7.5 years after correction, and another patient needed a subtalar fusion 6 months after correction. Both were conducted as an in situ fusion. As a rule, patients with malunions or nonunions after prior surgery had less favorable results than patients who had been treated nonoperatively. All patients, including the 1 patient needing a late ankle fusion, stated that given the same circumstances as preoperatively they would undergo corrective surgery again.

SUMMARY

Malunions and nonunions after central or peripheral fractures of the talar body are severe conditions for the affected patient, almost inevitably leading to pain and disability. Preoperative planning includes a thorough clinical and radiographic evaluation with assessment of the 3-dimensional outline of the malunion or nonunion, the amount of joint involvement, the presence of post-traumatic arthritis or infection, the extent of avascular necrosis, patient compliance, and relevant comorbidities. In properly selected, compliant patients without symptomatic arthritis or total AVN leading to collapse of the talar dome, and sufficient bone stock, secondary anatomic reconstruction with preservation of the essential peritalar joints may lead to considerable functional improvement. Bone grafting is needed after resection of a fibrous pseudarthrosis, sclerotic, or necrotic bone. Malunions and nonunions of the lateral or posterior process are treated adequately with excision of the malunited or loose fragments. If severe arthritis with full loss of cartilage is seen, corrective fusion of the affected joint(s) will still lead to alleviation of the symptoms and functional improvement.

REFERENCES

1. Zwipp H, Gavlik M, Rammelt S. Secondary anatomical reconstruction of malunited central talus fractures. Unfallchirurg 2014;117(9):767–75 [in German].
2. Canale ST, Kelly FB Jr. Fractures of the neck of the talus. J Bone Joint Surg Am 1978;60:143–56.

3. Inokuchi S, Ogawa K, Usami N. Classification of fractures of the talus: clear differentiation between neck and body fractures. Foot Ankle Int 1996;17(12): 748–50.

4. Rammelt S, Zwipp H. Talar neck and body fractures. Injury 2009;40(2):120–35.

5. Bibbo C, Anderson RB, Davis WH. Injury characteristics and the clinical outcome of subtalar dislocations: a clinical and radiographic analysis of 25 cases. Foot Ankle Int 2003;24(2):158–63.

6. Rammelt S, Goronzy J. Subtalar Dislocations. Foot Ankle Clin 2015;20(2): 253–64.

7. Rammelt S, Winkler J, Heineck J, et al. Anatomical reconstruction of malunited talus fractures: a prospective study of 10 patients followed for 4 years. Acta Orthop 2005;76(4):588–96.

8. Giuffrida AY, Lin SS, Abidi N, et al. Pseudo os trigonum sign: missed posteromedial talar facet fracture. Foot Ankle Int 2003;24(8):642–9.

9. Heckman JD, McLean MR. Fractures of the lateral process of the talus. Clin Orthop 1985;199:108–13.

10. Nyska M, Howard CB, Matan Y, et al. Fracture of the posterior body of the talus—the hidden fracture. Arch Orthop Trauma Surg 1998;117(1–2):114–7.

11. Rammelt S, Winkler J, Grass R, et al. Reconstruction after talar fractures. Foot Ankle Clin 2006;11(1):61–84, viii.

12. Mills HJ, Horne G. Fractures of the lateral process of the talus. Aust N Z J Surg 1987;57(9):643–6.

13. Sangeorzan BJ, Wagner UA, Harrington RM, et al. Contact characteristics of the subtalar joint: the effect of talar neck misalignment. J Orthop Res 1992;10(4): 544–51.

14. Lindvall E, Haidukewych G, DiPasquale T, et al. Open reduction and stable fixation of isolated, displaced talar neck and body fractures. J Bone Joint Surg Am 2004;86-A(10):2229–34.

15. Vallier HA, Nork SE, Benirschke SK, et al. Surgical treatment of talar body fractures. J Bone Joint Surg Am 2003;85-A(9):1716–24.

16. Thordarson DB, Triffon MJ, Terk MR. Magnetic resonance imaging to detect avascular necrosis after open reduction and internal fixation of talar neck fractures. Foot Ankle Int 1996;17(12):742–7.

17. Adelaar RS, Madrian JR. Avascular necrosis of the talus. Orthop Clin North Am 2004;35(3):383–95, xi.

18. Schuind F, Andrianne Y, Burny F, et al. Fractures et luxations de l'astragale. Revue de 359 cas. Acta Orthop Belg 1983;49(6):652–89.

19. Zwipp H, Rammelt S. Posttraumatic deformity correction at the foot. Zentralbl Chir 2003;128(3):218–26 [in German].

20. Langer P, Nickisch F, Spenciner D, et al. In vitro evaluation of the effect lateral process talar excision on ankle and subtalar joint stability. Foot Ankle Int 2007;28(1): 78–83.

21. Cronier P, Talha A, Massin P. Central talar fractures–therapeutic considerations. Injury 2004;35(Suppl 2):SB10–22.

22. Rammelt S, Zwipp H. Secondary correction of talar fractures: asking for trouble? Foot Ankle Int 2012;33(4):359–62.

23. Kim DH, Berkowitz MJ, Pressman DN. Avulsion fractures of the medial tubercle of the posterior process of the talus. Foot Ankle Int 2003;24(2):172–5.

24. Veazey BL, Heckman JD, Galindo MJ, et al. Excision of ununited fractures of the posterior process of the talus: a treatment for chronic posterior ankle pain. Foot Ankle 1992;13(8):453–7.

25. Asencio G, Rebai M, Bertin R, et al. Pseudarthrosis and non-union of disjunctive talar fractures. Rev Chir Orthop Reparatrice Appar Mot 2000;86(2):173–80 [in French].
26. Huang PJ, Cheng YM. Delayed surgical treatment for neglected or mal-reduced talar fractures. Int Orthop 2005;29(5):326–9.
27. Yu GR, Li B, Yang YF, et al. Surgical treatment of malunited or nonunited talus fractures. Zhonghua Wai Ke Za Zhi 2010;48(9):658–61 [in Chinese].
28. Barg A, Suter T, Nickisch F, et al. Osteotomies of the talar neck for posttraumatic malalignment. Foot Ankle Clin 2016, in press.

Joint-Preserving Osteotomies for Malaligned Intraarticular Calcaneal Fractures

 CrossMark

Stephen K. Benirschke, MD[a], Patricia A. Kramer, PhD[b],*

KEYWORDS

• Calcaneus • Subtalar joint • Osteotomy • Reconstruction

KEY POINTS

• Anatomic alignment of calcaneal fractures is imperative.
• Even with appropriate intervention, loss of reduction can occur.
• Anatomic reductions produce more and better options for subsequent reconstruction.
• Gastrocnemius recession is frequently necessary owing to inherent or acquired gastrocnemius equinus.

OSTEOTOMY IN CALCANEAL FRACTURES

Calcaneal osteotomies are indicated as salvage techniques to restore (some) function after failure or lack of definitive treatment for calcaneal fractures. These osteotomies can be used effectively to restore the gross shape of the calcaneus, which reorients the lateral hindfoot, and the relationship of the talus to the remainder of the tarsals and the tibia and fibula, which improves limb function. Nonetheless, the preferred option is always to appropriately treat calcaneal fractures acutely.

The need for calcaneal osteotomies can result from the initial conditions listed. We use the treatment of 7 patients to demonstrate the various challenges that arise owing to the complex nature of both the initial calcaneal injury and the subsequent salvage. Although all share the need to restore calcaneal morphology, the variety of techniques and nuances therein warrant detailed description.

The authors have nothing to disclose.
[a] Department of Orthopaedics and Sports Medicine, University of Washington, Seattle, Box 359798, WA 98195-9798, USA; [b] Department of Anthropology, University of Washington, Seattle, Box 353100, WA 98195-3100, USA
* Corresponding author.
E-mail address: pakramer@uw.edu

1. Conservative treatment of the initial injury. This situation is demonstrated for tongue variant calcaneal fractures by patient 1 (whose imaging is shown in **Fig. 1**) and for joint depression calcaneal fractures by patient 2 (**Fig. 2**).
2. Tongue variant fracture dislocations misdiagnosed on initial presentation. This is demonstrated by patient 3 (**Fig. 3**)
3. Open internal fixation without reduction. In these cases, the calcaneal fracture is appreciated and surgical invention occurs, but anatomic reduction of the calcaneus is not obtained. Patient 4 (**Fig. 4**) had a tongue variant fracture that was

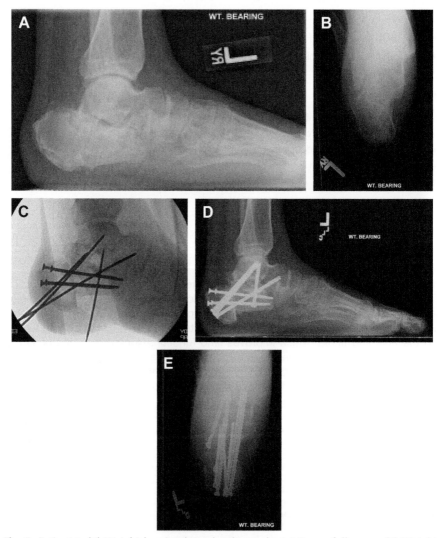

Fig. 1. Patient 1. (*A*) Weight-bearing lateral radiograph at 1.3-year follow-up. (*B*) Weight-bearing Harris axial radiograph at 1.3-year follow-up. (*C*) Intraoperative lateral radiograph with lateral wall tilting subtalar joint space and K-wires in place to act as guides for screws. (*D*) Weight-bearing lateral radiograph at 6-month follow-up. (*E*) Weight-bearing Harris axial radiograph at 6-month follow-up.

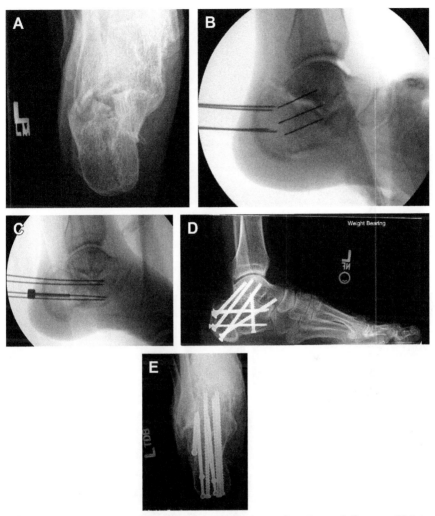

Fig. 2. Patient 2. (*A*) Weight-bearing Harris axial radiograph at 2-year follow-up. (*B*) Intra-operative lateral radiograph with 3 K-wires defining the osteotomy cut and 4 K-wires ready to secure tuber into new position. (*C*) Intraoperative lateral radiograph with a 2.5-mm drill sleeve ("top hat") in place over the K-wire. (*D*) Follow-up lateral radiograph. (*E*) Follow-up Harris axial radiograph. Note that osteotomy lag screws need to provide compression across the osteotomy, but that fusion screws (ie, positioning screws) should not provide compression across the subtalar joint to maintain calcaneal height.

salvageable without subtalar fusion, whereas patient 5 (**Fig. 5**) experienced a joint depression fracture and, owing to the deterioration of the posterior facet, required a subtalar fusion.

4. Calcaneal fractures from high-energy impacts with massive injury. In calcaneal fractures that include substantial posterior facet damage, collapse can be a likely sequelae of the initial injury. Patients 6 (**Fig. 6**) and 7 (**Fig. 7**) experienced different versions of this. Note that, despite the likelihood of calcaneal collapse, the initial definitive treatment of the calcaneal fracture is open reduction and internal fixation

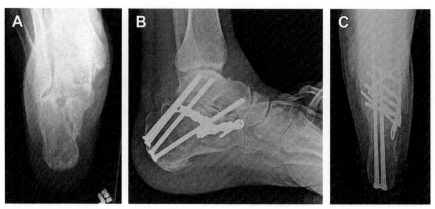

Fig. 3. Patient 3. (*A*) Injury Harris axial radiograph. (*B*) Intraoperative lateral radiograph. (*C*) Intraoperative Harris axial radiograph.

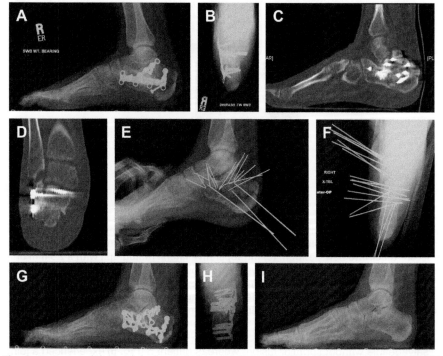

Fig. 4. Patient 4. (*A*) Simulated weight-bearing lateral radiograph after first surgery. (*B*) Simulated weight-bearing Harris axial radiograph after first surgery. (*C*) Sagittal plane computed tomography (CT) image. (*D*) Coronal plane CT image after first reduction. (*E*) Intraoperative lateral radiograph with multiple K-wires holding articular reduction in place. (*F*) Intraoperative Harris axial radiograph with K-wires. (*G*) The 6 month follow-up lateral radiograph. (*H*) The 6-month follow-up Harris axial radiograph. (*I*) Weight-bearing lateral radiograph taken 6 months before injury during treatment for a previous issue. Compare the preinjury lateral (*I*) with the follow-up view (*G*).

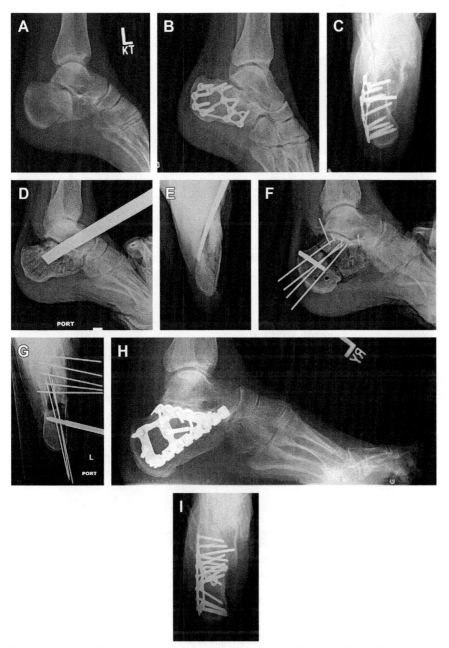

Fig. 5. Patient 5. (*A*) Injury lateral radiograph. (*B*) Lateral radiograph after initial reduction with plantar flexed foot. (*C*) Harris axial radiograph after initial reduction. (*D*) Intraoperative lateral radiograph shown with chisel used to osteotomize the malunited tuberosity and posterior facet. (*E*) Intraoperative Harris axial radiograph shown with chisel. (*F*) Intraoperative lateral radiograph. (*G*) Intraoperative Harris axial radiograph with Schanz pin used to restore tuberosity position. (*H*) Follow-up lateral radiograph. (*I*) Follow-up Harris axial radiograph.

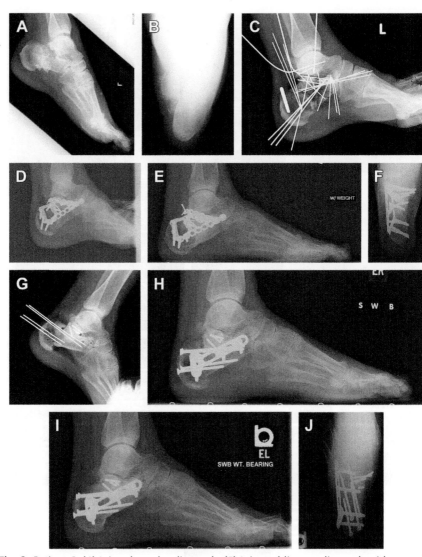

Fig. 6. Patient 6. (*A*) Injury lateral radiograph. (*B*) Injury oblique radiograph with posterior facet. (*C*) Intraoperative lateral radiograph with K-wires temporally securing small fragments. (*D*) Intraoperative lateral radiograph with fixation implants in place. (*E*) Intraoperative Harris axial radiograph. (*F*) Weight-bearing lateral radiograph with collapsed posterior facet. (*G*) Intraoperative lateral radiograph after osteotomy with K-wires in place. (*H*) Simulated weight-bearing lateral radiograph after osteotomy surgery. (*I*) Simulated weight-bearing lateral radiograph. (*J*) Simulated weight-bearing Harris axial radiograph.

for 2 reasons. First, it can be successful, ie, the fracture reduction is sometimes maintained, and second, anatomic initial reduction provides a more viable platform on which future salvage reconstructions can be undertaken.

Proper foot function depends on an anatomic hind foot (talus plus calcaneus). This includes a talus that is in proper relationship to the distal tibiofibular joint complex and to the navicular and also a calcaneus that supports the talus and the lateral midfoot.

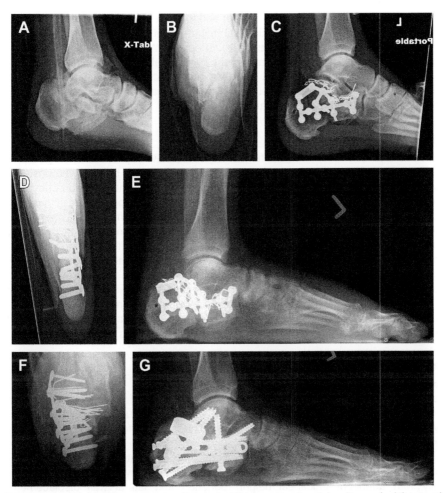

Fig. 7. Patient 7. (*A*) Injury lateral radiograph. (*B*) Injury Harris axial radiograph. (*C*) Lateral radiograph with definitive fixation in place. (*D*) Intraoperative Harris axial radiograph with definitive fixation in place. (*E*) The 4.5-month follow-up lateral radiograph with collapsed posterior facet. (*F*) The 4.5-month follow-up Harris axial radiograph with displaced tuberosity. (*G*) The 1-year follow-up lateral radiograph.

When the calcaneus is fractured, these critical relationships are disrupted. The posterior facet, which supports the talus, is often rotated and/or depressed (eg, see **Figs. 2**A and 5A, B) with lateral wall disruption (eg, see **Fig. 2**B). Additionally, the tuberosity can be translated laterally and rotated into varus (eg, see **Fig. 1**B) and the anterior process can be shortened and superiorly rotated (eg, see **Fig. 1**A). These displacements have the effect of reducing calcaneal height (through posterior facet depression and tuberosity rotation) and the relationship between the calcaneus and talus can be altered (eg, see **Fig. 1**A). Calcaneal length can be affected through anterior process shortening (eg, see **Fig. 1**A).

When these disruptions are not reduced anatomically, the change in calcaneal height and length and/or the orientation of the support for the talus changes the relationship between the midfoot and forefoot and the leg (eg, see **Fig. 1**D, E). When calcaneal length is not correct, the midfoot and forefoot can collapse laterally (lateral peritalar subluxation) and when calcaneal height is not correct, total limb length is shortened and anterior tibiotalar impingement occurs. When the posterior facet and anterior process are not in proper alignment, the talocalcaneal relationship is inadequate, producing acutely altered articular mechanics and, ultimately, subtalar arthrosis. A rotated tuberosity can alter heel strike mechanics. Consequently, restoration of calcaneal anatomy is imperative.

General Treatment Goals

With calcaneal fractures, treated either acutely or in a salvage procedure, the goal is to restore calcaneal height and length; to restore the relationship between the posterior facets of the calcaneus and of the talus and calcaneocuboid joint; and to properly align the tuberosity. The salvage of calcaneal malunions should be approached in much the same way as the primary treatment of calcaneal fractures: with meticulous attention to the soft tissues and to reducing the displaced fracture components to their preinjury anatomy.[1-3] Even in those cases where joint preservation is unlikely, anatomic reduction produces a better outcome than gross malalignment or malunion. Consequently, patients with grossly malunited calcaneal fractures should be considered as candidates for salvage procedures. In cases where the articular surface of the subtalar joint is intact, a joint-preserving osteotomy is the preferred procedure. The details of postoperative management have been described previously for calcaneal fractures and these techniques should be used for calcaneal osteotomies as well.

Treatment Details

Conservative initial treatment

Patients 1 and 2 were deliberately treated conservatively at the institution to which they initially presented, whereas patient 3 experienced an injury that was undetected by the medical personnel at the initial facility. The outcome for these scenarios was similar.

Patient 1 sustained a tongue variant calcaneal fracture that was treated conservatively at an outside facility even though the tongue fragment was displaced substantially with attendant calcaneal height reduction and lateral wall displacement. Weight-bearing lateral (see **Fig. 1**A) and Harris axial (see **Fig. 1**B) radiographic views from the outside facility obtained at the 1.3-year follow-up show that the tongue fragment from the initial injury remained evident. Patient 1 presented to our clinic approximately 2 years after injury with posttraumatic arthrosis, pain, and deformity from the injury and gastrocnemius equinus. He underwent a calcaneal osteotomy via an extensile lateral approach, as well as gastrocnemius and plantaris release and soleal fascia recession. Intraoperatively, the subtalar joint was distracted to establish height and restore sagittal hindfoot alignment orientation. After osteotomy of the posterior tuberosity, the tuber was moved distally, which required that the gastrocnemius lengthen. In the absence of a gastrocnemius recession, the distal positioning of the tuberosity is both difficult to obtain acutely and to maintain throughout the healing process. The position of the tuberosity relative to the posterior facet and anterior process was preserved with lag screws that compress across the osteotomy. The entire calcaneal complex was pinned to the talus with Kirschner-wires (K-wires). The subtalar joint space was then filled with lateral wall exostectomy, which was removed and shaped to fit the subtalar joint space (see **Fig. 1**C). The K-wires are used as guides for the 5.5-mm screws that secure the calcaneus to the talus. These positioning screws provide stability, but they do not compress across the joint to maintain the calcaneal height obtained via distraction. At the 1-year follow-up, the healed osteotomy's position is maintained during weight-bearing (see **Fig. 1**D, E).

Patient 2 sustained a joint depression calcaneal fracture that was treated conservatively at an outside facility. At the 1.3-year follow-up, the fracture lines are still clearly evident (see **Fig. 2**A) with a shortened length and displaced posterior facet compared with the uninjured foot. Intraoperatively, the 3 parallel K-wires that are perpendicular to the lateral surface of the calcaneus are used as guides to align the osteotomy blade and facilitate an accurate cut (see **Fig. 2**B). The plane of the osteotomy is of critical importance to establish the tuberosity orientation and calcaneal height. K-wires provide temporary support and are used as guides for definitive fixation (see **Fig. 2**C). K-wires are also used as guides for the screws used to obtain the subtalar fusion. After calcaneal osteotomy, anatomic position has been restored. At the 2-year follow-up, the osteotomy is healed and remodeled (see **Fig. 2**D, E).

Patient 3 sustained a tongue variant fracture dislocation that was misdiagnosed at an outside facility as an ankle sprain. The dislocation is subtle, but the Harris axial view clearly demonstrates the fracture and attendant dislocation (see **Fig. 3**A). After 4 months of progressive pain and repeat radiographs, computed tomography imaging at an outside facility demonstrated the fracture dislocation, and he was referred to our clinic for salvage of the malunion. The anatomy of the calcaneus was restored via osteotomy and a clipped Y-plate was used as a washer for the lag screws to compress the osteotomy plane. Owing to the degradation of the surface of the posterior facet from weight-bearing against the distal fibula, a subtalar fusion was also required at the time of the osteotomy (see **Fig. 3**B, C). At the 1-year follow up, the anatomic reduction has been maintained and the osteotomy and arthrodesis have progressed uneventfully.

Nonanatomic open reduction with fixation
Patients 1 through 3 reiterate the necessity of accurate initial assessment in emergency departments or by primary care physicians. Although foot morphology is complex, understanding the basic anatomy of the tarsals and metatarsals is a critical skill. Although patients 1 through 3 had injuries unrecognized by outside facilities, the injuries of patients 4 and 5 were detected and treated surgically, but the intraoperative reduction was not anatomic. Upon referral to our facility, the operative reduction was revised and new fixation used. One advantage that this scenario produces is that the patient is non–weight-bearing, so the calcaneus is not injured further, but, of course, the patient needs to undergo another operation.

Patient 4 sustained a tongue variant calcaneal fracture dislocation (similar to that of patient 3) that was treated surgically on the day of injury at an outside facility. When the skin flap created by the surgical approach became necrotic, she self-referred to our clinic. Although the radiographic views looked appropriate (see **Fig. 4**A, B), upon inspection of the computed tomography scans (see **Fig. 4**C, D), it was determined that the fracture had not been reduced adequately before the application of the internal fixation. Consequently, after debridement of the infected incisional wound, the calcaneal fragments were osteotomized and the reduction of the calcaneus was redone, using K-wires to secure the multiple calcaneal fragments (see **Fig. 4**E, F). She also required a gracilis free tissue transfer for coverage of her necrotic lateral wound. In this case, the posterior facet was salvageable. The follow-up images (see **Fig. 4**G, H) demonstrate that the new reduction was anatomic when compared with a radiograph obtained before the injury (as a comparison view for an orthopedic concern previously assessed in our clinic; see **Fig. 4**I).

Patient 5 sustained a joint depression injury (see **Fig. 5**A), with a substantially displaced posterior facet, that was treated initially at an outside facility. The internal fixation is applied with the posterior facet malreduced and the tuberosity in varus (see **Fig. 5**B, C), which is especially apparent when compared with the uninjured side. When the patient presented to our clinic at 1 year after the initial operation, the decision was made to redo the reduction, which required that the healed fracture fragments be osteotomized using a chisel (see **Fig. 5**D, E). Again, K-wires were used to secure the fragments (see **Fig. 5**F, G) after distraction and the restoration of height and before the definitive fixation was placed. Unfortunately, the posterior facet had been damaged substantially during the year of malalignment and patient 5 subsequently developed arthrosis and pain, even though the anatomic reduction was maintained (see **Fig. 5**H, I). A subtalar fusion was ultimately necessary.

Massive injury with anatomic open reduction

Patients 6 and 7 exemplify the philosophy that an anatomic reduction should always be the goal of reduction, even when the initial injury is substantial. In some cases, such as with patient 4, the calcaneus heals and the foot has good function after revision of the initial reduction, but even in cases like patient 5, an anatomic reduction facilitates the ultimately-required subtalar fusion with adequate foot function. This point is reiterated in the next pair of patients (6–7), for whom restoration of normal foot function was known to be unlikely from the initial treatment owing to the severity of the initial injury. Adequate function is possible, however, through careful attention to the surgical process.

Patient 6 sustained a medial open injury with a posteromedial extrusion of the entire posterior facet (see **Fig. 6**A, B). At reconstruction, multiple K-wires were used to hold the posterior facet in position (see **Fig. 6**C), until the definitive fixation was applied (see **Fig. 6**D). After 2 years, the posterior facet had collapsed into the calcaneal body (see **Fig. 6**E, F), although the other portions of the calcaneus have maintained their position when compared with the uninjured side. The osteotomy restored calcaneal height between the tuberosity and posterior facet (see **Fig. 6**G) and no subtalar fusion was required. Owing to the fragility of the bone fragments, a locking oblique T-plate is required to support the posterior facet (see **Fig. 6**H). At the 2-year follow-up, the osteotomy is consolidated firmly and the position of the foot has been maintained (see **Fig. 6**I, J).

Patient 7 sustained an injury that crushed the posterior facet (see **Fig. 7**A, B). This comminution required a series of wires to secure the small posterior facet fragments into place (see **Fig. 7**C, D). Compared with the uninjured side, an anatomic reduction was obtained, but it could not be maintained and collapsed occurred in the 6 months after surgery (see **Fig. 7**E, F). The subtalar arthrodesis procedure included distraction of the subtalar joint, and then fusion of the subtalar joint with the use of a tantalum insert to restore talar pitch. This intervention produced a functional foot, which, at 1 year follow-up (see **Fig. 7**G), had maintained the height and orientation created by the arthrodesis procedure.

SUMMARY

Joint-preserving osteotomies have been demonstrated to be effective at improving foot function. Rammelt and colleagues[4] reported that 5 patients with healed displaced intraarticular calcaneal fractures saw an improvement in average American Orthopaedic Foot and Ankle Society score from 19 to 81 after joint-preserving osteotomies, whereas Yu and colleagues[5] describe similar results in 24 patients. As these authors report and as we discuss, subtalar joint preservation is indicated if the articular cartilage is relatively undamaged. Weight-bearing on malaligned calcaneal fracture fragments can destroy the articular cartilage rapidly, which reiterates the necessity of treating displaced intraarticular calcaneal fractures with open reduction and anatomic internal reduction at the time of initial presentation.

Several key ideas emerge from these cases.

1. Anatomic reduction of calcaneal fractures with the restoration of the height and length of the entire calcaneus; of the position, relative to the talus, and shape of the posterior, middle, and anterior facets; and of the orientation of the heel and integrity of the lateral wall must be the first priority. Conservative treatment or misdiagnoses result in compromised foot function. Complex fractures patterns should be referred to specialists so that adequate reductions can be attempted.
2. Even with appropriate orthopedic intervention and care, some patients will not maintain their anatomic reductions and will need additional surgical intervention. In some cases, the initial injury is of such severity that the long-term prognosis for the reduction is bleak, although the senior author has had cases where the reduction of the calcaneus was maintained long term. In other cases, the etiology of the failure of the reduction is usually avascular collapse, potentially with associated insidious infection, even when physician and patient are committed to the treatment plan.
3. Even for injuries that have poor prognosis for maintenance of the reduction (and especially for those that have good prognosis), operative reduction and internal fixation is required, because an anatomic reduction allows the salvage procedure to be less complicated with a greater chance for long-term maintenance of the correction and good foot function. When anatomic reductions fail, they tend to do so via a collapse of the posterior facet into the calcaneal body. This is potentially owing to the low trabecular density inferior to the angle of Gissane, but more likely owing to a failure of the posterior facet to revascularize and unite with the tuberosity posteriorly, the sustentaculum medially and the anterior process anteriorly. The osteotomy, then, reestablishes height, but orientation is grossly intact and does not need adjustment.
4. When the posterior facet joint surface is intact, realignment of the calcaneus via a joint-preserving osteotomy produces a foot that functions relatively normally. The subtalar joint can be preserved and function restored as long as the articular cartilage has not been (further) damaged by bearing weight on a malaligned joint surface. Typically, the critical window of opportunity is 6 months.
5. Gastrocnemius equinus (either inherent in the patient or caused by prolonged splinting with the foot in a plantar flexion position) inhibits the ability of the surgeon to obtain anatomic reduction and can put fragile reductions at risk of failure owing to the pull of the Achilles tendon on the calcaneal tuberosity and pressure of an equinus forefoot on subtalar joint reconstruction. Consequently, assessment of gastrocnemius equinus and recession of the gastrocnemius if equinus is present is necessary.

REFERENCES

1. Benirschke SK, Kramer PA. Fractures of the calcaneus. Orthopaedic Knowledge Online Journal 2003. Available at: http://orthoportal.aaos.org/oko/.
2. Benirschke SK, Kramer PA. Wound healing complications in closed and open calcaneal fractures. J Orthop Trauma 2004;18:1–6.
3. Benirschke SK, Kramer PA. Hot topic: update on the management of calcaneal fractures. Orthopaedic Knowledge Online Journal 2012. Available at: http://orthoportal.aaos.org/oko/.

4. Rammelt S, Grass R, Zwipp H. Joint-preserving osteotomy for malunited intra-articular calcaneal fractures. J Orthop Trauma 2013;27:234–8.
5. Yu GR, Hu SJ, Yang YF, et al. Reconstruction of calcaneal fracture malunion with osteotomy and subtalar joint salvage: technique and outcomes. Foot Ankle Int 2013;34:726–33.

Corrective Osteotomies for Malunited Tongue-Type Calcaneal Fractures

Guang-Rong Yu, MD*, Ming-Zhu Zhang, MD, PhD,
Yun-Feng Yang, MD

KEYWORDS

- Calcaneal malunion • Corrective osteotomy • Joint preserving • Foot biomechanics

KEY POINTS

- If most of the cartilage cover at the posterior calcaneal facet is viable based on direct evaluation, the subtalar joint can be preserved by corrective osteotomy.
- The goal of surgery is to restore the height, width, and length of the calcaneus. Abnormal Gissane and Böhler angles, a collapsed arch, posterior facet tilt, and incongruity should be corrected.
- For complete depression of posterior facet, an opening wedge osteotomy is performed to reconstruct the joint, and restore the height and Gissane and Böhler angles.
- For multiple levels of depression, osteotomy should be performed in different levels; additional insertion of a bone graft can correct an external tilt of the posterior facet and support the restored calcaneal height.
- A closing wedge osteotomy at the calcaneal sulcus can correct varus deformity.

INTRODUCTION

The optimal treatment of calcaneus fractures remains controversial.[1–3] Conservative treatment of displaced calcaneal fractures and inadequate reduction and fixation or failed surgery may lead to symptomatic calcaneal malunions.[4–6] The calcaneus supports the talus and its position in relation to the ground and determines the appropriate position of the articular surface of the talus with the tibia. Surface incongruity of the posterior subtalar joint facet results in painful posttraumatic arthritis.[7–9] The lateral calcaneal wall expansion results in heel widening with associated subfibular impingement causing peroneal stenosis, tendinitis, or dislocation.[10] The decrease in calcaneal body height results in loss of the talar declination, which results in anterior tibiotalar

The authors have nothing to disclose.
Department of Orthopedics, Tongji Hospital, School of Medicine, Tongji University, 389 Xincun Road, Shanghai 200065, China
* Corresponding author.
E-mail address: yuguangrong@hotmail.com

Foot Ankle Clin N Am 21 (2016) 123–134
http://dx.doi.org/10.1016/j.fcl.2015.09.005
1083-7515/16/$ – see front matter © 2016 Elsevier Inc. All rights reserved.

impingement and decreased ankle dorsiflexion.[11,12] Therefore, the function of the ankle, subtalar, and transverse tarsal joints can all be affected, leading to pain and disability. The tongue-type is one of the typical calcaneal fracture patterns. Besides involving the previously mentioned characteristics, a malunited calcaneal tuberosity fracture can result in hindfoot malalignment.[13]

The subtalar joint is crucial for normal foot and ankle function. When the subtalar joint is fused, mobility of the adjacent joints increases to compensate for the loss of subtalar joint function. Abduction and adduction of the foot decreases by 50% following subtalar arthrodesis.[14] Among others, Savory and colleagues[15] found that isolated subtalar arthrodesis reduces talonavicular joint function. Consequently, the subtalar joint should be preserved if possible. For planning the correction of calcaneal malunions it is important to assess the deformity and the subtalar joint condition.

INDICATIONS FOR CORRECTIVE OSTEOTOMY OF TONGUE-TYPE FRACTURES

Corrective osteotomy of tongue-type fractures is indicated when the subtalar joint condition is good enough to preserve in young patients, the primary injury is within 1 year, and the damaged cartilage area is less than 30% in young patients and 50% in patients more than 60 years old. Malunited Sanders type IIa, IIb, IIc, and IIIac fractures can be corrected by osteotomy if the previously mentioned criteria are fulfilled.

For malunited Sanders type IIIbc and IV fractures, the cartilage damage usually is beyond repair and reconstruction is difficult. Therefore, corrective arthrodesis is usually required for those cases. Cartilage damage is assessed by radiograph (**Fig. 1**), computed tomography (CT), MRI (**Fig. 2**), and most importantly by direct inspection with distraction of the joint. This article describes the technique to correct malunited tongue-type calcaneal fracture by osteotomies.

The cause of malunited tongue fractures is improper treatment by either nonoperative or failed operative methods. It is important to realize that the corrective surgery of calcaneal malunions is very demanding and should only be performed by surgeons with a vast expertise in hindfoot surgery. The price of error is usually disability.

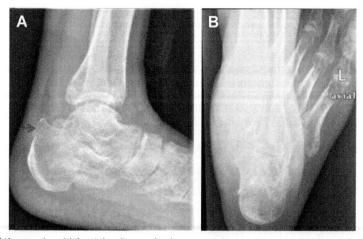

Fig. 1. (A) Lateral and (B) axial radiographs demonstrating a tongue-type calcaneal malunion. The arrow shows a posttraumatic Haglund deformity.

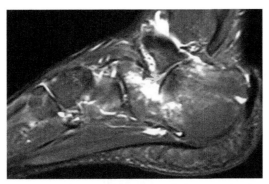

Fig. 2. MRI demonstrates complete cartilage cover of the posterior facet of the calcaneus with viable cartilage (*arrow*).

CALCANEAL MALUNION CLASSIFICATIONS

Stephens and Sanders[6] developed a classification system for calcaneal malunions based on coronal CT scans. This system is based solely on coronal images; thus, it does not address hindfoot height or talar declination.

Zwipp and Rammelt[5] developed a classification system to guide surgical management of calcaneal malunions (**Table 1**). This classification highlights the potential issues that may exist after traumatic injury, although deformities may fit more than one type. All malunions without subtalar arthritis (ie, those amenable for joint-preserving corrections) are collectively termed "type 0."[2]

Those two classifications do not specifically address malunited tongue-type fractures. Based our experience, these can be classified into two types and four subtypes (**Table 2**).

PREOPERATIVE PLANNING
Clinical Evaluation

Calcaneal fracture malunion severely affects the global function of the foot and ankle, eventually leading to pain and permanent disability. The evaluation for revision surgery begins with a thorough clinical evaluation of the factors that contribute to patient dissatisfaction, functional impairment, and pain. Clinical evaluation includes the inspection for hindfoot deformity, alignment, foot arch, heel widening, ankle, subtalar, and midtarsal joint mobility, and limb length. Frequently, the malunited calcaneal fracture involves some form of peroneal tendon pathology, such as impingement,

Table 1	
Zwipp and Rammelt classification of calcaneal malunions	
Type	**Characteristics**
1	Subtalar incongruency, normal calcaneal morphology
2	Additional heel varus or valgus
3	Additional loss of hindfoot height
4	Additional lateral translation of the calcaneal tuberosity
5	Additional talar tilt or dorsiflexion past neutral

From Zwipp H, Rammelt S. Posttraumatic deformity correction at the foot. Zentralbl Chir 2003;128(3):221; with permission.

Table 2	
Tongue-type calcaneal malunion classification	
Type	Characteristics
I	Depression of the whole tongue fragment
1A	Subtalar congruency with anterior rotation of the tongue fragment (**Fig. 3**A)
1B	Subtalar incongruency with anterior rotation of the tongue fragment (**Fig. 4**A)
1C	Subtalar incongruency with anterior rotation and external tilt of the tongue fragment (**Fig. 5**A, C)
II	Posterior facet depression in different levels (**Fig. 6**A, B)

subluxation, or dislocation, because of the lateral wall blowout or lateral dislocation of the tuberosity. An altered and poorly tolerated gait pattern results from varus malunion of the calcaneal tuberosity.

Patients with a calcaneal varus deformity usually complain about lateral ankle instability or pain, sometimes also medial ankle joint pain. Physical examination reveals a hindfoot varus deformity with a medially prominent heel while the patient is standing. Ankle joint dorsiflexion is limited by tibiotalar exostosis or impingement secondary to an abnormal talar tilt resulting from a loss of heel height. Frequently, the subtalar joint remains stiff following a joint depression injury. Ankle instability is checked with the anterior drawer and talar tilt tests clinically and radiographically. Gait examination may also reveal abnormalities with weakened push-off strength.

Radiographic Evaluation

Weight-bearing radiographs are crucial for the evaluation of calcaneal malunions. A lateral radiograph can reveal the degree of joint depression and its morphology (see **Fig. 1**). Loss of calcaneal body height, as represented by a decreased Böhler angle, results in collapse of the arch and a more horizontal talus, which leads to anterior tibiotalar impingement and limitation of ankle dorsiflexion. A posttraumatic Haglund deformity with a prominent posterior tuberosity is often seen in malunited tongue-type fractures. The surgeon also needs to evaluate the position of the calcaneal tuberosity on a standing hindfoot alignment view. The axial view or Saltzman view can show

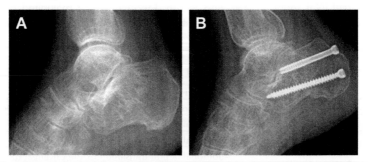

Fig. 3. Type IA maluinon. (*A*) Lateral radiograph showing depression the whole posterior facet. The subtalar joint becomes congruent with anterior rotation of the tongue fragment. (*B*) Postoperative radiograph demonstrates anatomic reconstruction maintained with two screws.

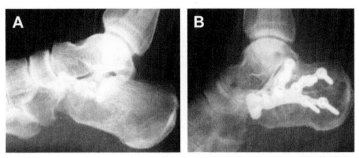

Fig. 4. Type IB maluinon. (*A*) Lateral radiograph showing depression of the whole posterior facet. The subtalar joint remains incongruent with anterior rotation of the tongue fragment. (*B*) Postoperative radiograph demonstrates anatomic reconstruction maintained with a lateral calcaneal plate.

abnormal alignment, calcaneal widening, subtalar tilt, and impingement. The calcaneal tuberosity can be significantly malaligned in varus or valgus along with being translated medially or laterally. The contralateral side is used as a control if unaffected. Standing anteroposterior ankle views determine if adaptive ankle joint deformity lateral ankle or calcaneofibular impingement is present. Stress lateral radiographs are obtained if lateral ankle instability is suspected.

CT scanning is generally used to evaluate calcaneal malunions given the irregular anatomy of the calcaneus, to determine the extent of subtalar joint arthritis, and to obtain a three-dimensional view through reconstructions for surgical planning. Stephens and Sanders[6] and Zwipp and Rammelt[5] classified calcaneal malunions based on CT scans and provided treatment recommendations. CT scanning is especially useful to evaluate joint depression and angulation (see **Figs. 5**C and **6**B). Any preoperative planning of corrective osteotomies should be based on CT images.

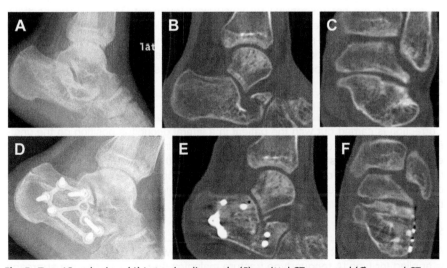

Fig. 5. Type IC malunion. (*A*) Lateral radiograph, (*B*) sagittal CT scan, and (*C*) coronal CT scan show depression of the whole posterior facet. The subtalar joint is incongruent with anterior rotation and external tilt of the tongue fragment. (*D*) Postoperative radiograph, (*E*) sagittal CT scan, and (*F*) coronal CT scan demonstrate anatomic reduction of the calcaneus.

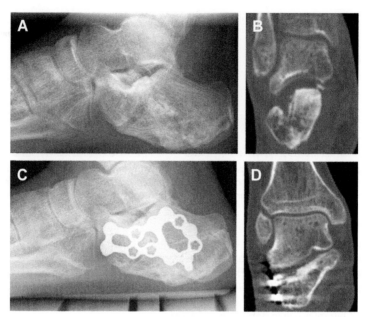

Fig. 6. Type II malunion. (*A*) Lateral radiograph and (*B*) coronal CT scan show collapse of the posterior facet at different levels. (*C*) Postoperative radiograph and (*D*) CT scan demonstrate anatomic reduction of the subtalar joint after calcaneal osteotomies and plate fixation.

MRI is more sensitive for cartilage viability and osteonecrosis (see **Fig. 2**). It may therefore be helpful for treatment decision making. Ligament and tendon conditions are also evaluated by MRI.

Surgical management of calcaneal malunion should be reserved for active, healthy patients who are not responsive to nonsurgical treatment. The following sections discuss the four subtypes of tongue fracture deformities that are encountered and surgical options for joint-preserving calcaneal osteotomies to further improve the patient's morphology, gait, and functional abilities. At times, the surgeon has to assess the patient on multiple occasions to determine the best suited procedures before performing surgery.

Patient Positioning

Correction is carried out with the patient in a lateral decubitus position on the unaffected side. It is our preference to use a regular operating room table with a radiolucent end to allow surgeons to more comfortably stand at the end of the table. A bolster is made to support the operative extremity and the other leg is extended to move the contralateral foot out of the radiographic field. A tourniquet is applied to the ipsilateral thigh.

Surgical Approach

An oblique incision at the calcaneal sulcus just below the course of the sural nerve is applied for type IA tongue-type fracture malunion (**Fig. 7**). This oblique approach adds minimal soft tissue injury and has a low risk of wound complications. The subtalar joint is inspected and the osteotomy performed with this approach (**Fig. 8**A).

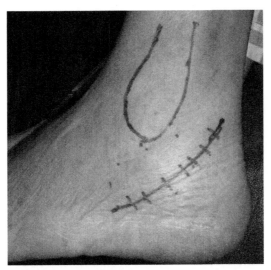

Fig. 7. The same patient in **Fig. 3**. An oblique incision at the calcaneal sulcus is applied for type IA tongue malunion just below the course of the sural nerve.

For other type of tongue malunion fractures except type IA, an extended lateral approach is used as described previously (**Fig. 9**).[16,17] The subtalar joint is exposed and cleared of fibrous adhesions. The cartilage status of the posterior facet of the talus and calcaneus is assessed. The osteotomy is performed carefully with thin saw and wide chisels along the former fractures as analyzed with the preoperative CT scans. It is uncommon to be unable to close the wound if surgery is directed at restoring hindfoot anatomy and biomechanics, but occasionally this does occur. Under these circumstances it is important not to apply any tension to the wound margins. The reconstruction has to be taken down and a more modest correction obtained. Patients are warned preoperatively of the possibility that the reconstruction may be performed in a staged manner.

SURGICAL PROCEDURE

The full-thickness subperiosteal flap of the extensile lateral approach to the calcaneus is raised. Care is taken to avoid injury to inferior branches of the superficial peroneal nerve and superior branches of the sural nerve. The calcaneofibular ligament is cut to access the posterior subtalar joint.

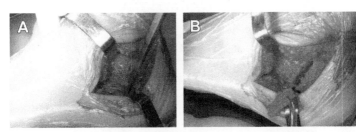

Fig. 8. (*A*) A closing wedge osteotomy is performed to correct varus deformity. (*B*) An oblique osteotomy is performed. An opening wedge osteotomy can correct the varus deformity.

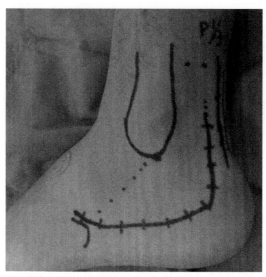

Fig. 9. The landmarks of the extended lateral approach are outlined with skin marker.

Removal of Hardware (Revision Surgery)

Before performing a calcaneal osteotomy to correct a residual deformity, any surgical hardware may need to be removed if it prevents osteotomy. The implants are removed through the original incision.

Excision of the Lateral Wall

A significant amount of pain typically results from the lateral wall exostosis and subsequent peroneal tendon pathology. We perform a lateral wall exostectomy for subfibular impingement and/or associated peroneal pathology, such as tendinopathy, dislocation, or stenosis.

The lateral calcaneal wall is exposed and excised to a more normal width by using a wide chisel or thin-bladed osteotomy saw, starting posteriorly with a slight medial angulation relative to the longitudinal axis of the calcaneus, leaving more residual bone plantarly (**Fig. 10**). The lateral wall should be aligned with the lateral process of the talus after excision. The peroneal tendons are freed from adhesions and decompressed below the tip of the lateral malleolus. The excised lateral wall fragment is

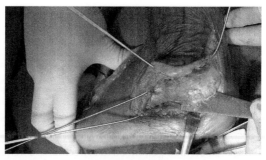

Fig. 10. Lateral wall exostosectomy with a wide chisel.

retained, and shaped to appropriate size for later use as a bone-block graft. A small distractor is applied to expose the subtalar joint through two 2.5-mm K-wires that are placed into the talar and calcaneal tuberosity (**Fig. 11**).

The peroneal tendons are elevated in their sheath and retracted by another K-wire. Adequate dissection is done until complete visualization of the posterior facet is accomplished.

Osteotomy

The osteotomy is based on the malunion type. In type 1A, vertical or oblique osteotomy is performed and the tuberosity translated downward about 1.0 cm depending on the individual Böhler angle (**Fig. 8B**). A pelvic reduction forceps or 3.5-mm Steinmann pin is used to reduce the displaced fragment. Angulation should be corrected at the same time.

For type 1B lateral horizontal osteotomy is performed to elevate the depressed joint fragment (**Fig. 12**). The joint surface collapse, calcaneal height, Böhler and Gissane angles, and subtalar congruency should be restored. For type 1C, in addition to the horizontal osteotomy as performed for type IB malunions, lateral elevation of the joint fragment is added. This opening wedge can correct the external tilt (**Fig. 13A**). A bone graft is placed beneath to elevate the fragment (**Fig. 13B**). The bone graft is usually obtained from the lateral wall excision. If this is not enough, autologous iliac crest bone or allograft is used.

In type 2, osteotomies are performed under the depressed steps to restore the joint surface. Bone grafts are placed to fill the space below the joint and support correction. Intraoperative fluoroscopic images including Brodén projections should be obtained to verify the joint reconstruction after osteotomy and bone grafting. The subtalar joint is inspected directly (**Fig. 14**).

If hindfoot varus is greater than 5°, a vertical closing wedge osteotomy is performed at the calcaneal sulcus. If a valgus deformity exits, an opening wedge osteotomy should be carried out. If there is a posttraumatic Haglund deformity, the bony prominence should be excised.

After osteotomies and bone grafting, K-wires are used for temporary fixation. The alignment and morphology of the calcaneus is verified under C-arm fluoroscopy. The fragments are fixed with plate or/and screws.

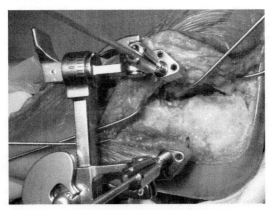

Fig. 11. A foot distractor (Depuy-Synthes) is applied to explore the subtalar joint. The cartilage condition is inspected and probed directly.

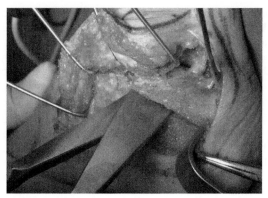

Fig. 12. A lateral horizontal osteotomy is performed to elevate the depressed joint.

POSTOPERATIVE CARE

Postoperatively, patients are put in a lower leg splint for 7 to 10 days. Elevation of the operated foot for 24 hours is usual. Early range of motion exercises of the ankle and subtalar joints are started out of the splint on the second day after surgery. A suction drainage is usually used to prevent a postoperative hematoma that may require revision. If drainage is less than 20 mL per day, the tube can be removed. The patient is mobilized non-weight-bearing until the wound has healed and until bone healing is sufficient, as verified by CT scans, to allow a progressive load-bearing. Partial weight-bearing is allowed in an air cast walker boot after 6 weeks. Weight-bearing should be gradually increased after radiographic evidence of bony union at 10 to 12 weeks. Patients are seen for follow-up at 6 weeks, 3 months, 6 months, 1 year, and 2 years.

RESULTS

A total of 45 patients (45 feet) were treated in by our group, 24 of which have been reported previously.[16] The American Orthopaedic Foot and Ankle Society ankle and hindfoot score at 1 year follow-up was 82.8 (range, 79.5–89.3) as compared with 62.4 (range, 48.2–71.6) before reconstruction. Radiographs showed that Böhler angle, Gissane angle, talus declination angle, and width and height of calcaneus were improved. Heng and Kwon[13] reported an operative technique for percutaneous osteotomy of 6 weeks delayed tongue-type calcaneus fractures. This approach is not suitable for the patients from our series, which presented about 8 months after

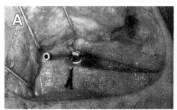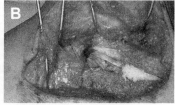

Fig. 13. (*A*) The joint is elevated laterally more than medially to correct the tilt of the fragment. A vertical closing wedge osteotomy is used to correct calcaneal varus deformity. (*B*) A bone wedge from the excised lateral wall is placed beneath the joint-bearing fragment to restore the joint anatomy and calcaneal height.

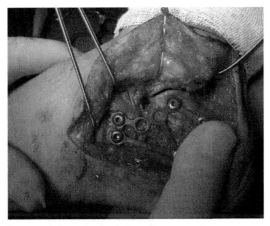

Fig. 14. Direct inspection of the subtalar joint after correction.

the initial fracture. Rammelt and colleagues[17] performed intra-articular osteotomies to preserve the subtalar joint in a different manner, with good results. We here present a method specific only for tongue-type malunited calcaneal fractures.

SUMMARY

Symptomatic calcaneal malunion results from the pathoanatomy that disrupts the normal relationship of the hindfoot and its function. The malunion leads to disability and pain for the affected patients. Corrective surgery is the only option in these cases. Subtalar arthrodesis is required in most severe deformities. But if the calcaneal posterior facet morphology and subtalar joint cartilage is of sufficient quality, especially in young patients, the joint could be preserved. Different methods are used for correction based on the classification of the malunion. A thorough preoperative planning and elaborate surgical technique is the key to restore the anatomy of the calcaneus. Adequate postoperative care and rehabilitation are crucial for regaining hindfoot function.

REFERENCES

1. Buckley R, Tough S, McCormack R, et al. Operative compared with nonoperative treatment of displaced intra-articular calcaneal fractures: a prospective, randomized, controlled multicenter trial. J Bone Joint Surg Am 2002;84-A(10):1733–44.
2. Rammelt S, Zwipp H. Fractures of the calcaneus: current treatment strategies. Acta Chir Orthop Traumatol Cech 2014;81(3):177–96.
3. Agren PH, Wretenberg P, Sayed-Noor AS. Operative versus nonoperative treatment of displaced intra-articular calcaneal fractures: a prospective, randomized, controlled multicenter trial. J Bone Joint Surg Am 2013;95(15):1351–7.
4. Lim EV, Leung JP. Complications of intraarticular calcaneal fractures. Clin Orthop Relat Res 2001;(391):7–16.
5. Zwipp H, Rammelt S. Posttraumatic deformity correction at the foot. Zentralbl Chir 2003;128(3):218–26 [in German].
6. Stephens HM, Sanders R. Calcaneal malunions: results of a prognostic computed tomography classification system. Foot Ankle Int 1996;17(7):395–401.

7. Sanders R, Vaupel ZM, Erdogan M, et al. Operative treatment of displaced intra-articular calcaneal fractures: long-term (10-20 years) results in 108 fractures using a prognostic CT classification. J Orthop Trauma 2014;28(10):551–63.
8. Griffin D, Parsons N, Shaw E, et al. Operative versus non-operative treatment for closed, displaced, intra-articular fractures of the calcaneus: randomised controlled trial. BMJ 2014;349:g4483.
9. Fan WL, Sun HZ, Wu SY, et al. Subtalar distraction osteogenesis for posttraumatic arthritis following intra-articular calcaneal fractures. Foot Ankle Int 2013;34(3): 398–402.
10. Yoshimura I, Ichimura R, Kanazawa K, et al. Simultaneous use of lateral calcaneal ostectomy and subtalar arthroscopic debridement for residual pain after a calcaneal fracture. J Foot Ankle Surg 2015;54(1):37–40.
11. Reddy V, Fukuda T, Ptaszek AJ. Calcaneus malunion and nonunion. Foot Ankle Clin 2007;12(1):125–35.
12. Banerjee R, Saltzman C, Anderson RB, et al. Management of calcaneal malunion. J Am Acad Orthop Surg 2011;19(1):27–36.
13. Heng M, Kwon JY. Percutaneous osteotomy for irreducible or malunited tongue-type calcaneus fractures. Foot Ankle Int 2014;35(4):408–14.
14. Mann RA, Baumgarten M. Subtalar fusion for isolated subtalar disorders. Preliminary report. Clin Orthop Relat Res 1988;(226):260–5.
15. Savory KM, Wülker N, Stukenborg C, et al. Biomechanics of the hindfoot joints in response to degenerative hindfoot arthrodeses. Clin Biomech (Bristol, Avon) 1998;13(1):62–70.
16. Yu GR, Hu SJ, Yang YF, et al. Reconstruction of calcaneal fracture malunion with osteotomy and subtalar joint salvage: technique and outcomes. Foot Ankle Int 2013;34(5):726–33.
17. Rammelt S, Grass R, Zwipp H. Joint-preserving osteotomy for malunited intra-articular calcaneal fractures. J Orthop Trauma 2013;27(10):e234–8.

Corrective Osteotomies for Malunited Extra-Articular Calcaneal Fractures

 CrossMark

John Ketz, MD[a],*, Michael Clare, MD[b], Roy Sanders, MD[b]

KEYWORDS

• Calcaneal malunion • Extra-articular correction • Joint preserving
• Chronic peroneals dislocation • Exostectomy

KEY POINTS

- Correction of calcaneal malunions is a technically difficult procedure that carries many risks for the patient.
- Joint-sparing extra-articular procedures for calcaneal malunions should be carefully evaluated, as few will be amenable to this approach.
- The presence of articular malunion or arthritic change to the subtalar joint is a contraindication for a joint-sparing approach.
- Simple exostectomy or osteotomy procedures can be effective at relieving localized pain caused by excessive pressure from plantar and posterior tuberosity protuberances.
- Associated soft tissue issues should be considered before proceeding with surgery, including skin and soft tissue quality, chronically dislocated peroneals tendons, and equinus contracture.

INTRODUCTION

Calcaneal fractures are the most common fracture of the hindfoot. These fractures often produce a high level of dysfunction.[1,2] Historically, most fractures were treated conservatively because of lack of knowledge concerning the injury.[3–5] However, as that method of treatment produced unacceptable results, alternative interventions were investigated. Currently, many surgical options exist for the treatment of calcaneal fractures, including external fixation, percutaneous techniques, and open reduction internal fixation either through a traditional extensile lateral or sinus tarsi approach.[6–10] Conservative or poor surgical techniques continue to produce calcaneal malunions. Calcaneal malunions present a difficult scenario for the treating orthopedic surgeon and can lead to deformity and rapid, progressive arthrosis of the subtalar joint.

The authors have nothing to disclose.
[a] Department of Orthopaedic Surgery, University of Rochester, 601 Elmwood Ave., Box 665, Rochester, NY 14642, USA; [b] University of South Florida Department of Orthopaedic Surgery, Florida Orthopaedic Institute, 13020 Telecom Parkway North, Tampa, FL 33637, USA
* Corresponding author.
E-mail address: john_ketz@urmc.rochester.edu

Foot Ankle Clin N Am 21 (2016) 135–145
http://dx.doi.org/10.1016/j.fcl.2015.09.006
1083-7515/16/$ – see front matter © 2016 Elsevier Inc. All rights reserved.

foot.theclinics.com

PATHOLOGY AND DEFORMITY EVALUATION

Most calcaneal fractures involve the posterior facet and only approximately 25% are extra-articular fractures.[11] Many deformities are created as a result of the injury (**Fig. 1**). Despite the joint being preserved in these injuries, the deformities that arise can present issues for the patient in the future. An axial force can cause the talus to be driven into the calcaneus through the neutral triangle, which is an area of relative osteopenia. The bone collapses and pushes out the lateral wall of the calcaneus. The lateral wall displacement or *blow out* creates subfibular impingement. This displacement causes lateral pain most noted with uneven surfaces. With impaction of the talus into the calcaneus, there is decreased talar declination angle caused by the depression of the talar body into the fracture, creating anterior ankle impingement. Fractures through the body of the calcaneus can also create shortening of the calcaneus. The subsequent varus deformity of the posterior tuberosity causes patients to ambulate through the lateral border of the foot. It also creates stiffness as the medial column stiffens with hindfoot varus. Fractures of the posterior tuberosity of the calcaneus can create posterior prominence of the tuberosity leading to discomfort from direct pressure.

CLASSIFICATION

Currently, 2 classification systems for calcaneal malunions exist. The Stephens and Sanders classification system places the malunion into 3 categories.[12] Type I involves mild subtalar arthrosis with subfibular impingement, which can be treated with simple exostectomy. Type II malunions have advanced arthrosis with subfibular impingement. In addition to exostectomy, subtalar arthrodesis is advocated for these types of deformities. The type III deformity adds hindfoot varus to the previous deformities. This deformity requires corrective calcaneal osteotomy in addition to fusion and exostectomy. This classification system has merits in that it is prognostic and helps to guide the surgeon with treatment. However, this classification does not address anterior ankle impingement from talar body collapse.

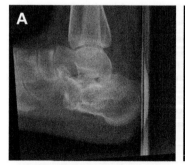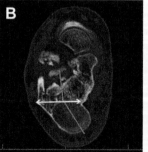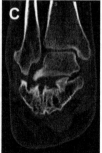

Fig. 1. (*A*) Lateral weight-bearing radiograph of a 23-year-old woman shows a calcaneal malunion with loss of height and Böhler's angle. Also, note the subsidence of the talus into the calcaneus creating anterior ankle impingement. (*B*) Axial view of the CT scan shows expansion of the lateral wall (*arrow*) and the severe varus angulation of the posterior tuberosity with shortening. (*C*) Semicoronal view of the CT scan shows subfibular impingement and subtalar arthrosis. Note the presence of the healed distal fibular avulsion fracture from injury to the superior peroneals retinaculum suggestive of chronic peroneal dislocation.

Zwipp and Rammelt[13] and Rammelt and Zwipp[14] described a classification system based on the progressive deformities associated with calcaneal malunions. Type 0 has deformity without evidence of arthrosis. Type I has joint arthrosis without deformity. Type II has additional varus deformity coupled with joint incongruity or arthrosis. Type III deformities account for the loss of height creating anterior ankle impingement. Type IV involves lateral and superior migration of the lateral wall fragment. Type V involves incongruity of the ankle mortise caused by impaction of the talus into the calcaneus. Each of these types is further subcategorized by pathology. Subgroup A is a solid malunion, B is a pseudoarthrosis, and C has avascular necrosis with collapse.

Indications and Preoperative Evaluation

Once advanced arthrosis has occurred at the subtalar joint, arthrodesis is the most reliable method of treatment with combined procedures to correct any existing deformities. This occurs in most calcaneal malunions. However, in select cases, joint-sparing procedures can restore the anatomic alignment of the calcaneus while avoiding sacrificing the subtalar joint and function. For Zwipp and Rammelt type 0 and Stephens and Sanders type I malunions, this is the preferred method.[12,14] This can be done using extra-articular osteotomies and intra-articular osteotomies or a combination of both.

These are technically challenging procedures, and proper patient selection is crucial. The patient's soft tissue envelope and neurovascular status should be well inspected. Proper patient postoperative compliance is paramount to avoiding complications. If uninjured, evaluation of the patients' contralateral limb will help guide the surgeon in restoring normal alignment. Soft tissue contractures, particularly equinus contractures, should be assessed, as patients may also require soft tissue releases in addition to boney procedures. The peroneal tendons should also be evaluated, as they can be chronically dislocated as a result of the initial injury.

Imaging

Weight-bearing radiographs of the foot and ankle can give the surgeon better understanding of the foot position under loading conditions. These radiographs can be dramatically different compared with non–weight-bearing radiographs. The lateral view will show loss of height (Böhler's angle) and the presence of anterior ankle impingement. The Harris axial heel image shows the presence and extent of hindfoot varus. Broden views, if performed well, will show the subtalar joint incongruity, if present. This can typically also be seen on the ankle mortise image. Computed tomography (CT) scan is extremely useful in evaluating deformity, as it depicts the deformity in a 3-dimensional fashion. CT scan provides important information on the arthritic status of the subtalar and calcaneocuboid joints and whether a nonunion is present. Added information includes the presence of subfibular impingement and evaluation of the subtalar joint. However, the status of the cartilage and decision for arthrodesis is best evaluated intraoperatively under direct evaluation.

TREATMENT
Conservative Treatment

Conservative care is typically difficult in patients with calcaneal deformities because often there is shortening with loss of height and gait disturbances. The deformities and injury also create significant stiffness of the subtalar joint and, to a lesser degree, the ankle joint. Rest, ice, anti-inflammatories, orthotics, and activity modification are the main treatment options. Orthotics can range from University of California Biomechanics Laboratory shoe inserts to more advanced bracing options such as an *Ankle Foot Orthosis* or Arizona style brace. Conservative care should be reserved for poor surgical candidates either because of medical comorbidities or a poor soft tissue envelope.

OPERATIVE CARE
Lateral Wall Exostectomy

For Stevens and Sanders type I deformities in which there is subfibular impingement because of lateral wall expansion, a lateral wall exostectomy can be beneficial. This was described by Cotton initially.[15] Care must be taken to remove only the lateral wall and not to enter the subtalar joint. There is typically a significant amount of bone that is removed, and this can be used as autologous bone graft for a nonunion (Zwipp subgroup B) or for adjunctive subtalar fusion if the joint is arthritic. After removal of the bone, the peroneal tendons should be inspected and evaluated for frank dislocation or instability, as the lateral wall exostosis can often push the tendons laterally such that the superior peroneal retinaculum becomes insufficient (**Fig. 2**).

Technique

The patient is positioned in the lateral decubitus position, and an extensile lateral incision is used. Subperiosteal dissection is performed using a "no-touch" technique on the lateral flap. Once the flap is elevated, it is retracted with 1.6-mm K-wires placed into the distal fibula, talar neck, and cuboid. Using a large osteotomy saw blade the lateral wall is resected. The saw blade should be slightly angled medially to the

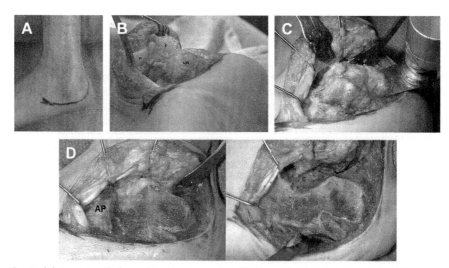

Fig. 2. (*A*) An extensile lateral incision is made with the patient in the lateral decubitus position. (*B*) Subperiosteal dissection is performed and the lateral wall (LW) and the peroneals tendons (P) are exposed. Note the presence of subfibular impingement caused by the proximity of the tip of the fibula (F) to the lateral wall. (*C*) The lateral wall is then removed with large sagittal saw. Retractors are placed to prevent injury to the joint and distal fibula. K-wires have been placed to protect the flap and the peroneals tendons. (*D*) The lateral wall is removed exposing the joint (*left*). The saw is then used to remove any lateral expansion from the anterior process (AP) (*right*). After resection, the angle of Gissane can then be appreciated.

longitudinal axis of the calcaneus. Care should be taken to avoid penetration into the talofibular joint and the subtalar joint. If there is some mild lateral arthrosis of the subtalar joint, it can also be resected without destabilizing the joint.

The exostectomy is also carried out distally to remove extruded bone lateral to the calcaneocuboid joint. If done correctly the exostectomy will be removed en bloc with an osteotome. If it is to be used with an adjunct procedure for autograft, it is protected on the back table for later use. At this point, after removal of the bone, attention should be turned to the undersurface of the flap. A Freer elevator is passed into the peroneal sheath, and then the integrity of the retinaculum is tested at the level of the distal fibula. If there is instability, the vertical limb of the incision should be extended, and the superior peroneal retinaculum should be reconstructed to the posterolateral aspect of the fibula using either a "pants over vest" technique or with suture anchors (**Fig. 3**). Alternatively, this technique can be done through a separate smaller incision over the posterolateral aspect of the fibula, if the soft tissues allow (**Fig. 4**). Closure is performed over a drain using meticulous technique in a 3-layered fashion.

Excessive Plantar Bone

Because of the axial force creating the fracture, there may be bone fragments that are pushed plantar to the calcaneus. During the healing process, these may continue to grow, creating a painful prominence on the plantar aspect of the foot. These fragments may be removed through an incision made using the longitudinal limb of the extensile approach. Because of scarring and the multiple plantar soft tissue attachment, this bone can often be difficult to remove. A plantar incision should be avoided, if possible, because of the morbidity associated with incisions on the sole of the foot (**Fig. 5**).

A   **B**

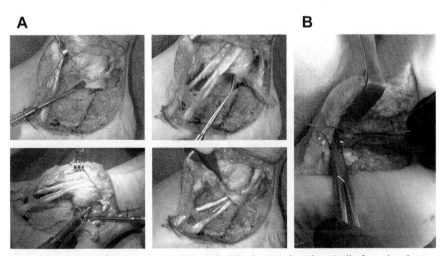

Fig. 3. (*A*) The superficial peroneal retinaculum is dissected and typically found to be torn from the posterolateral aspect of the fibula (*top left*). The fibular groove is inspected and debrided to allow for reduction of the tendons (*top right*). If needed, the fibular groove can be deepened with the use of a burr (*bottom right*). The tendons are then reduced into their anatomic position, and the retinaculum is repaired to the posterolateral aspect of the fibula. (*B*) Two suture anchors are placed into the posterolateral aspect of the fibula, and the retinaculum is directly repaired to the fibula. Imbrication of the superficial peroneal retinaculum can be performed if needed.

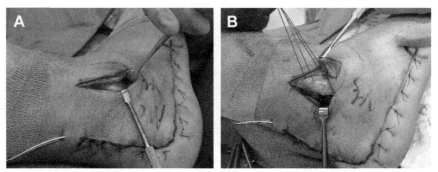

Fig. 4. (*A*) After closure of the extensile lateral flap, a small posterolateral incision is made over the fibula. The superficial peroneal retinaculum is incised, and the peroneal groove is debrided before tendon reduction. (*B*) Similarly, 2 anchors are placed into the fibula and the superficial peroneal retinaculum is repaired.

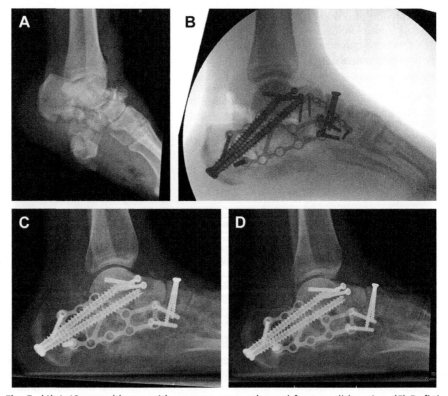

Fig. 5. (*A*) A 19-year-old man with a severe open calcaneal fracture dislocation. (*B*) Definitive fixation was performed of his multiple fractures and primary arthrodesis of his subtalar and calcaneocuboid joint. (*C*) At 1 year, the patient had a painful plantar exostosis that developed during healing of his injury. (*D*) The patient underwent simple plantar exostectomy that alleviated his plantar symptoms.

Posterior Tuberosity Osteotomy

Posterior heel pain can occur owing to conservatively or operatively treated fractures because of superior migration of the posterior tuberosity.[16] This migration is most commonly seen in tongue type fractures in which the tuberosity remains superior and potentially posteriorly translated, which causes direct pressure against shoes and can be a significant pain generator. Similar to the lateral wall osteotomy, this can be removed and produce pain relief for the patient. The main factor determining the approach is based on the size and extent of the fragment. If the fragment is small or mostly laterally based, a lateral-based approach can be used and the fragment can be removed without significantly disrupting the Achilles tendon. However, if the fragment is large and is thought to contain a significant amount of Achilles insertion, a direct posterior approach should be taken with an Achilles central tendon splitting technique. This technique creates adequate visualization for removal of the exostosis while allowing for direct Achilles tendon repair or reinsertion. With this type of malunion, careful evaluation should be done for gastrosoleus contractures. Often some form of lengthening should accompany this procedure.

In scenarios in which the Achilles insertion is entirely attached to the malunited fragment, a complete osteotomy with rigid fixation must be performed to reduce and restore the anatomy. Care should be taken to avoid residual posterior heel bossing, and lengthening of the gastrosoleus complex is needed before correction of the deformity (**Fig. 6**).

Lateral Technique (Smaller Exostoses)

The patient is placed in the lateral position and a posterolateral incision is made adjacent to the tendon. Care should be taken to avoid the sural neurovascular structures. The deep fascia and lateral tendon fibers are split longitudinally. From this incision the superior Achilles is dissected from the boney exostosis and protected with retractors. A microsagittal saw is then used to cut the prominent bone. The bone resection is then removed using osteotomes. The tissue layers are then closed in layered fashion.

Posterior Technique (Larger Exostoses)

The patient is placed in the prone position. A direct midline incision is made over the Achilles tendon. A longitudinal incision is made through the paratenon and Achilles tendon. The tendon is then dissected medially and laterally off of the superior posterior

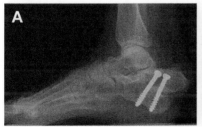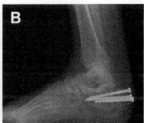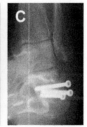

Fig. 6. (*A, B*) Extra-articular deformity of a 40-year-old patient 1 year after fracture of the calcaneal tuberosity. The patient complains of a shoe pain at the back edge of the deformed heel and overload of the sole as a result of the reduced contact surface. (*C*) The corrective osteotomy follows the former fracture line and restores the shape of the calcaneal body; thus, the physiologic hindfoot is restored with pain relief. (*From* Rammelt S, Schneiders W, Zwipp H. Joint-preserving osteotomy for calcaneal malunions. Unfallchirurg 2014;117(9):776–84; with permission.)

tuberosity. With the bone exposed and tendon edges retracted, a microsagittal saw is used to remove the bone. The bed of the tendon is then prepared with a burr to create a bleeding surface and 2 suture anchors are placed in the insertion site. One limb from each suture anchor is used to repair the midline split, and the remaining limbs are used to repair the bed to the insertion site. The soft tissues are then closed in layered fashion (**Fig. 7**).

Postoperative Care

After both lateral, inferior, and posterior exostectomies, the patient is kept non–weight bearing in a splint for 2 weeks. They are then placed into a weight-bearing fracture

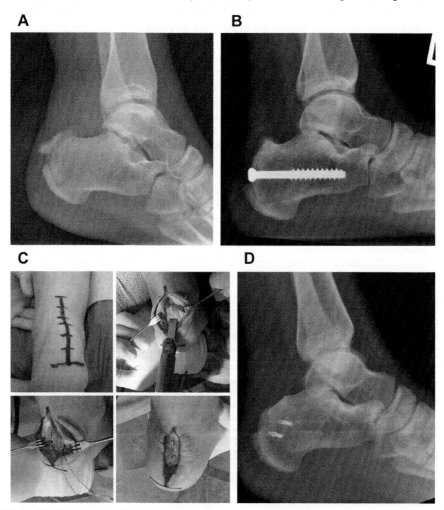

Fig. 7. (*A, B*) A 39-year-old woman who sustained a posterior tuberosity fracture was treated with screw fixation and had a painful posterior prominence over the heel. (*C*) A midline posterior incision is made directly over the Achilles tendon (*top left*). The Achilles is incised longitudinally to expose the posterior tuberosity prominence, which is then removed with a microsagittal saw (*top right*). Two suture anchors are then placed at the insertion site to repair the tendon back to the bone (*bottom left and right*). (*D*) Postoperative radiographs show excision of the painful prominence with suture anchor repair of the Achilles tendon.

boot and begin range-of-motion exercises based on the stability of the wound. If a great deal of Achilles tendon dissection was performed from the posterior approach or a tuberosity osteotomy was performed, prolonged immobilization with protected weight bearing is needed in the fracture boot for 6 to 8 weeks with heel lifts.

Lateral Calcaneal Osteotomy

Fractures through the body of the calcaneus can affect the overall architecture of the calcaneus. With any loss of the medial osseous structures, the hindfoot forces the posterior tuberosity into varus and migrates superiorly. The varus created can produce significant symptoms. These symptoms can be treated with osteotomies through the posterior tuberosity. A Dwyer osteotomy is a closing lateral wedge osteotomy. This technique effectively restores valgus alignment to the hindfoot. However, it can lead to further shortening of the calcaneus. Consideration can be given to this osteotomy if there is adequate length of the body with only a varus deformity. For shortening with varus, a lateral displacing calcaneal osteotomy can be performed. If there is excessive shortening, either a tricortical allograft or autograft can be used to add length.

Technique

Because many of these patients will also have lateral exostoses that will require excision, the patient is placed into the lateral decubitus position. An extensile lateral incision is used, and, if needed, the lateral wall exostectomy is performed as described above. At this point, the calcaneal osteotomy is marked using fluoroscopic guidance, and the osteotomy is performed with a thin-blade large oscillating saw. The osteotomy is completed with a large osteotome and the soft tissue attachments are freed with dissection. The osteotomy is then translated laterally to correct the varus alignment and held temporarily with a K-wire. If there is excessive shortening of the calcaneus, an autologous graft (lateral exostectomy) can be used as well as an allograft. The osteotomy site is then secured by the placement of 2 screws. The size of the screws should be determined based on the size and anatomy of the patient (**Fig. 8**).

Postoperative Care

After calcaneal osteotomy, the patient is kept non–weight bearing in a splint for 2 weeks. Once the wound is healed, the patient can be placed into a fracture boot, and ankle range-of-motion exercises may begin. The patient may begin progressive

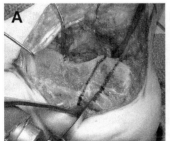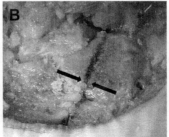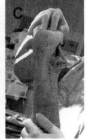

Fig. 8. (*A*) Using an extensile lateral incision, the lateral wall and posterior tuberosity of the calcaneus is exposed. A Dwyer osteotomy is marked and completed with a large oscillating saw. (*B*) Once the osteotomy is completed, it is mobilized and the compressed (shown by the *arrows*), correcting the hindfoot varus. It is then stabilized with large partially threaded cannulated screws. (*C*) Intraoperative inspection shows adequate restoration of normal hindfoot valgus.

weight bearing at 6 weeks in the fracture walker boot. The boot is then discontinued at 10 weeks with gradual return to activities.

RESULTS

Because most patients present with advanced subtalar arthrosis, there are limited studies evaluating the results of extra-articular joint-sparing procedures for correction of calcaneal malunions. Braly and colleagues[17] reported on a group of 19 patients who underwent lateral decompression with peroneal tenolysis/repair for calcaneal malunions. In 11 of those patients, the procedure was done as an alternative to subtalar fusion, with 9 patients having satisfactory results. Stephens and Sanders[12] prospectively followed up with 26 malunions in 7 patients with type I deformities. Of those 7 patients, 6 had excellent and 1 had good results using the modified Maryland Foot Score.

SUMMARY

The most effective way to treat calcaneal malunions is avoidance. With any articular fracture, progressive arthrosis and dysfunction are common. By restoring the anatomy initially through reduction, late reconstructive options become less complicated. Numerous studies have shown that restoration of the anatomic alignment either through percutaneous or open techniques is effective. In patients with no or minimal articular degeneration, extra-articular joint-sparing procedures can be performed. This represents a small select group who may benefit from simple osteotomy procedures with associated soft tissue reconstruction, if needed.

REFERENCES

1. Sangeorzan BJ, Hansen ST Jr. Early and late posttraumatic foot reconstruction. Clin Orthop Relat Res 1989;243:86–91.
2. Sanders R. Displaced intra-articular fractures of the calcaneus. J Bone Joint Surg Am 2000;82:225–50.
3. Lindsay WR, Dewar FP. Fractures of the os calcis. Am J Surg 1958;95(4):555–76.
4. Conn HR. The treatment of fractures of the os calcis. J Bone Joint Surg Am 1935; 17:392–405.
5. Pozo JL, Kirwan EO, Jackson AM. The long-term results of conservative management of severely displaced fractures of the calcaneus. J Bone Joint Surg Br 1984; 66(3):386–90.
6. Essex-Lopresti P. The mechanism, reduction technique, and results in fractures of the os calcis. Br J Surg 1952;39(157):395–419.
7. Sanders R, Fortin P, DiPasquale T, et al. Operative treatment in 120 displaced intraarticular calcaneal fractures. Results using a prognostic computed tomography scan classification. Clin Orthop Relat Res 1993;(290):87–95.
8. Tornetta P 3rd. The Essex-Lopresti reduction for calcaneal fractures revisited. J Orthop Trauma 1998;12(7):469–73.
9. Rammelt S, Amlang M, Barthel S, et al. Percutaneous treatment of less severe intraarticular calcaneal fractures. Clin Orthop Relat Res 2010;468(4):983–90.
10. Kline AJ, Anderson RB, Davis WH, et al. Minimally invasive technique versus an extensile lateral approach for intra-articular calcaneal fractures. Foot Ankle Int 2013;34(0):773–80.
11. Zwipp H, Rammelt S, Barthel S. Calcaneal fractures–open reduction and internal fixation (ORIF). Injury 2004;35(Suppl 2):SB46–54.

12. Stephens HM, Sanders R. Calcaneal malunions: results of a prognostic computed tomography classification system. Foot Ankle Int 1996;17(7):395–401.

13. Zwipp H, Rammelt S. Posttraumatische Korrekturoperationen am Fuß. Zentralbl Chir 2003;128(3):218–26.

14. Rammelt S, Zwipp H. Corrective arthrodeses and osteotomies for post-traumatic hindfoot malalignment: indications, techniques, results. Int Orthop 2013;37(9): 1707–17.

15. Cotton FJ. Old os calcis fractures. Ann Surg 1921;74:294–303.

16. Squires B, Allen PE, Livingstone J, et al. Fractures of the tuberosity of the calcaneus. J Bone Joint Surg Br 2001;83(1):55–61.

17. Braly WG, Bishop JO, Tullos HS. Lateral decompression for malunited os calcis fractures. Foot Ankle 1985;6(2):90–6.

Joint-Sparing Corrections of Malunited Chopart Joint Injuries

Wolfgang Schneiders, MD, PhD, Stefan Rammelt, MD, PhD*

KEYWORDS

- Chopart joint • Midtarsal joint • Malunion • Nonunion • Correction • Osteotomy

KEY POINTS

- Typical findings of malunited Chopart injuries include shortening of the medial or lateral foot column leading to forefoot adduction or abduction, cavus or flat foot deformities, and joint incongruities rapidly leading to posttraumatic arthritis.
- The aim of correction is axial realignment of the midfoot to the hindfoot while limiting fusion to the affected joint or joints.
- Joint-preserving corrections are generally possible for all 4 bony components of the Chopart joint to restore normal foot function but only in carefully selected compliant patients with sufficient bone stock and cartilage quality.
- For patients with symptomatic posttraumatic arthritis, presence of avascular necrosis or infection, severe comorbidities, poor soft tissue conditions, or poor bone stock, arthrodesis with realignment and bone grafting remains the treatment of choice.

INTRODUCTION

Injuries to the midtarsal (Chopart) joint are frequently overlooked or misinterpreted and, therefore, not treated adequately at initial presentation.[1] The reasons include their relatively low incidence, the wide variance of the clinical presentation, and the lack of knowledge about the main radiographic projections and pathognomonic signs.[2–4] It is estimated that up to 40% of Chopart fracture-dislocations are either dismissed as midfoot sprains or misjudged as isolated fractures and, therefore, treated inadequately.[5–8] Due to its location and functional importance, loss of joint congruity and stability in the midtarsal region jeopardizes the global foot function. Bony malunion at the Chopart joint regularly leads to painful malunion or nonunion with a

The authors have nothing to disclose.
University Center for Orthopaedics & Traumatology, University Hospital Carl Gustav Carus at the TU Dresden, Fetscherstrasse 74, Dresden 01307, Germany
* Corresponding author.
E-mail address: strammelt@hotmail.com

3-dimensional deformity, residual instability, and a rapid progression of posttraumatic arthritis.[9] The main salvage procedure for these severe conditions is corrective fusion of the affected joint or joints with axial realignment of the foot.[2,10] This article reviews the indications, techniques, and results of joint-preserving corrective surgery for Chopart malunion and nonunion based on a simple classification.

ANATOMY AND PATHOMECHANICS OF ACUTE INJURIES

The Chopart joint (ie, midtarsal joint, transverse tarsal joint) consists of 2 separate joints that are closely interrelated. At the level of the Chopart joint, the length of the medial column of the foot is maintained by the integrity of the talar head and the navicular, the length of the lateral column by the anterior process of the calcaneus and the cuboid.[7] The more flexible talonavicular joint belongs to the talocalcaneonavicular joint (coxa pedis) that is essential for normal foot function.[11] It allows a 3-dimensional movement of the midfoot and forefoot with respect to the ankle and hindfoot, that is, eversion and inversion of the whole foot.[12,13] The calcaneocuboid joint has less range of motion.[13–15] It is, however, important for maintaining flexibility of the lateral column, which has only 2 joints, whereas the medial column has 3. Both joints act as a unit in allowing the forefoot to pivot relative to the hindfoot about the longitudinal axis of the foot, describing a screw-like motion[12] and contributing to the total eversion and inversion movements.

In their landmark paper, Main and Jowett[5] analyzed the mechanism in 71 acute injuries to the Chopart joint. Longitudinal forces were responsible for 40% of the injuries. Forced adduction of the forefoot during the impact led to medial stress and fractures to the tarsal navicular and/or talar head. Forced abduction of the forefoot during the impact led to lateral stress and fractures to the anterior process of the calcaneus and/or the cuboid (Fig. 1). Rotatory forces resulted in additional deformity (swivel dislocation). Less frequently, plantar forces and crush injuries with irregular fracture patterns were seen.[5] Considering the mechanism of injury, with every compression fracture on the medial side, a distractive force resulting in either a fracture, avulsion, or ligament rupture has to be suspected on the lateral side, and vice versa.[7,16] Zwipp,[17] therefore, presented a descriptive classification related to the site of bony injury. The fractures and dislocations at the Chopart joint are termed (1) purely transligamentous, (2) transtalar, (3) transcalcaneal, (4) transnavicular, (5) transcuboidal, and (6) combinations of (2) to (5). Almost half of all Chopart joint injuries involve at least 2 bones and the distal ones are more frequently affected than the proximal ones.[7]

PATHOANATOMY OF POSTTRAUMATIC DEFORMITIES

It follows directly from the injury mechanism that a typical deformity after transtalar or transnavicular fractures not treated adequately is shortening of the medial column. Subsequent varus malalignment of the hindfoot, midfoot cavus, and forefoot adduction results in a 3-dimensional deformity.[1] Malunion of transcalcaneal or transcuboidal fractures will result in shortening of the lateral column of the foot with hindfoot valgus, collapse of the medial arch at the midfoot, and forefoot abduction. Plantar or dorsal dislocation of the tarsal bones from vertical or axial forces results in a flat foot or cavus deformity. Additional rotatory (swivel) malalignment will lead to marked inversion or eversion with chronic subluxation. In many cases, a combination of these components will be seen, resulting in complex deformities. Malfunction due to malalignment of 1 midtarsal joint will considerably decrease motion, not only in the other midtarsal joint,

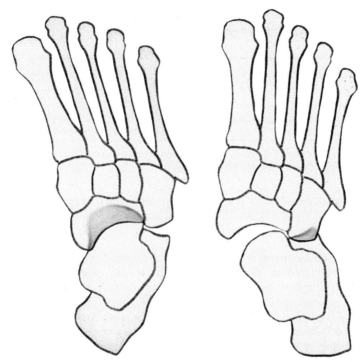

Fig. 1. Mechanism of injury at the Chopart joint according to Main and Jowett,[5] 1975, with forced abduction and adduction of the forefoot and midfoot with respect to the hindfoot. (*From* Rammelt S, Grass R, Schikore H, et al. Verletzungen des Chopart-Gelenks. Unfallchirurg 2002;105(4):374; with permission.)

but also in the neighboring joints, especially the subtalar joint, significantly affecting global foot function.[13–15]

Due to the high and eccentric loading, especially of the talonavicular joint, any posttraumatic incongruity will rapidly lead to irreversible cartilage damage. During simulated normal gait with a ground reaction force of 350 Nm, intra-articular forces at the talonavicular and calcaneocuboid joint reach values of 174 N/149 N and a peak pressure of 3877 kPa/3396 kPa, respectively.[18] Therefore, at the time of presentation, most cases will already have progressed to posttraumatic arthritis, making corrective fusion of the affected joint or joints the treatment of choice.[2,7,9,10]

PRINCIPLES OF TREATMENT

Surgical correction of malunion and nonunion at the Chopart joint aims at axial realignment of the midfoot and forefoot to the ankle and hindfoot with rebalancing the lateral and medial column of the foot.[1,10,19,20] Recently, a classification of posttraumatic deformities at the midtarsal joint was proposed to provide a rationale for surgical reconstruction (**Table 1**).

In type I and II deformities, a joint-preserving reconstruction can be considered. Solid malunion (type I) is treated with corrective osteotomies and secondary internal fixation after realignment (**Figs. 2–6**). Bone grafting is mostly needed to regain length of the medial or lateral column. Cases with isolated nonunion (type II) can be treated with debridement, bone grafting, and joint-sparing fixation (**Figs. 7** and **8**).

Table 1 Classification of posttraumatic deformities at the midtarsal joint	
Type	**Pathologic Condition**
I	Joint incongruity
II	Nonunion
III	I or II with arthritis at the calcaneocuboid joint
IV	I or II with arthritis at the talonavicular joint
V	Bilateral arthritis and complex deformity

From Rammelt S, Thielemann F, Zwipp H. Reconstruction of malunited Chopart fracture-dislocations. FussSprungg 2009;7:107; with permission.

Specifically the tarsal navicular and, to a lesser extent, the talar head are susceptible to focal avascular necrosis (AVN). Patients have to be instructed preoperatively about the risk of development or progression of the AVN after any corrective procedure.

In types III and IV, correction of the deformity is followed by fusion of the obviously arthritic joint. Nonetheless, the other joint can be spared, which will be of particular benefit in type III deformities in which salvage of the talonavicular joint is feasible (**Figs. 9–12**).

Patients with bilateral arthritis and complex deformities (type V) are treated with realignment and fusion of the talonavicular and calcaneocuboid joints.[1,20] In cases of long-standing, complex deformities with arthritis of adjacent joints, extensile bone loss, or AVN, fusion has to be extended to the subtalar joint (resulting in corrective triple fusion) or the naviculocuneiform joints.[2,5,7]

INDICATIONS AND CONTRAINDICATIONS

Joint-sparing corrections of Chopart joint malunion or nonunion are indicated in the absence of posttraumatic arthritis in young, active, and compliant patients. Contraindications include relevant comorbidities such as poorly controlled diabetes mellitus, manifest neuropathy, severe neurovascular deficits, ongoing infection, substance abuse, and immunodeficiency.

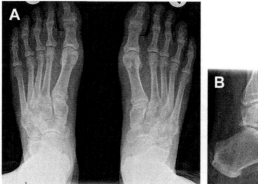
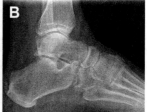

Fig. 2. (*A, B*) Weightbearing radiographs of a 59-year-old man presenting with a painful malunion 5 months after an overlooked transcuboidal Chopart fracture-dislocation (type I deformity).

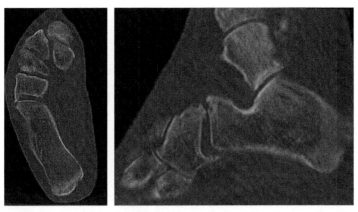

Fig. 3. CT scans showing impression of the joint surface to the calcaneocuboid joint (same patient as in **Fig. 2**, see article for details).

PATIENT ASSESSMENT AND PREOPERATIVE PLANNING

Patients with midfoot malunion and nonunion are evaluated clinically with respect to pain, activities, and functional demands; restrictions in daily life; gross deformities; soft tissue conditions (eg, scars, callosities); neurovascular status; and active or passive range of motion and stability at the ankle, subtalar, and midtarsal joints.

Radiographic analysis of the deformity includes standard anteroposterior (dorso-plantar) and lateral weightbearing radiographs of both feet as well as a 45° oblique view (see **Fig. 2**). Computed tomography (CT) scans are mandatory for determining the joint status, the 3-dimensional outline of the deformity, and the exact amount of

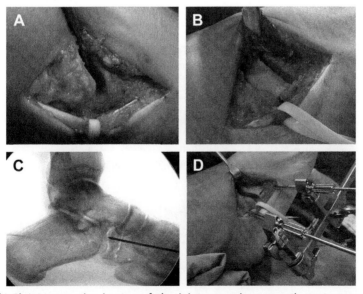

Fig. 4. (*A-D*) Intraoperative images of the joint-preserving corrective osteotomy of the cuboid using the resected lateral wall as a bone graft (same patient as in **Figs. 2** and **3**, see article for details).

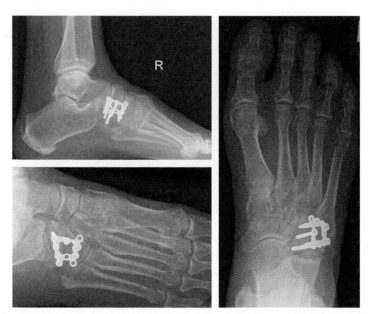

Fig. 5. Standing and oblique radiographs 1 year after correction and fixation of the cuboid with an interlocking plate showing bony union and anatomic alignment (same patient as in **Figs. 2–4**, see article for details).

any nonunion (see **Fig. 3**). If there is any suspicion of AVN in these investigations, an MRI should be performed to confirm its presence and to determine its size. Routine C-reactive protein levels and leukocyte counts are obtained to rule out infection. The decision whether to reconstruct or fuse the affected joints will frequently be made at the time of surgery, after direct inspection and probing of the cartilage (see **Figs.** 4A, 8B

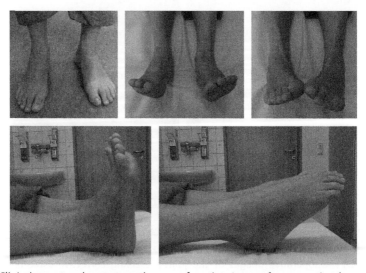

Fig. 6. Clinical aspect and near-normal range of motion 1 year after correction (same patient as in **Figs. 2–5**, see article for details).

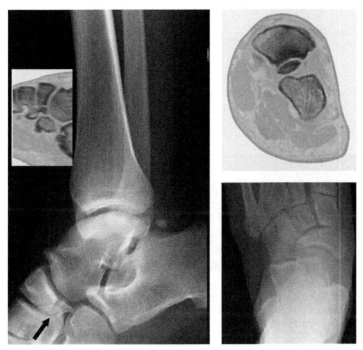

Fig. 7. Radiographs and CT scans of a 24-year-old man presenting with a painful nonunion of the navicular (type II deformity) 11 months after an overlooked transnavicular Chopart fracture-dislocation in a traffic accident with multiple injuries. Nonunion of the plantar aspect of the navicular is detected (*arrow*).

and **11A**). The patient is instructed that a fusion of the talonavicular or calcaneocuboid joint is carried out if manifest arthritis with substantial loss of the cartilage is detected intraoperatively. Furthermore, the risk of the development or progression of posttraumatic arthritis in case of a joint-preserving procedure is critically discussed.[1]

SURGICAL APPROACHES

The patient is placed in a supine position with a tourniquet on the thigh. A bump is placed beneath the ipsilateral hip to avoid external rotation of the leg. The talonavicular joint is approached by a longitudinal anteromedial or midline incision over the midfoot, depending on the site of the malunited fracture or nonunion. The approach requires careful dissection of the subcutaneous tissues and protection of the intermediate dorsal cutaneous nerve, a branch of the superficial peroneal nerve. After opening the fascia and incising the inferior extensor retinacula, the deep neurovascular bundle consisting of the dorsalis pedis artery and deep peroneal nerve is gently mobilized laterally together with the extensor digitorum longus tendon.[1,11] If the lateral aspect of the navicular has to be exposed, both tendon and neurovascular bundle are retracted medially and held away with a soft strap. The approach should extend from the talar neck proximally to the naviculocuneiform joints distally. To obtain an adequate exposure of the spherical joint surface, a small distractor is placed between the talar neck and the medial cuneiform.[19]

The calcaneocuboid joint is accessed via an anterolateral approach.[19] The incision is oblique and lies directly above the peroneal tendons. It starts at the sinus tarsi and

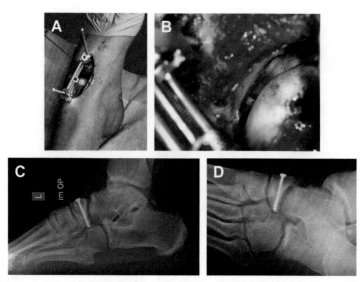

Fig. 8. (*A*) To view the plantar aspect of the spherical joint, a mini-distractor was placed between the talar neck and the navicular. (*B*) Direct inspection shows the nonunion but no signs of posttraumatic arthritis. (*C*) Correction included debridement, bone grafting, and screw fixation. (*D*) Solid union is seen after 3 months (same patient as in **Fig. 7**, see article for details).

extends to the fifth tarsometatarsal joint. The length of the incision should be reasonably generous to avoid excessive traction on the wound margins with subsequent skin necrosis.[2] Care has to be taken to not injure the sural nerve in the subcutaneous tissue, especially with severe scarring. The peroneal tendons are identified, gently mobilized plantarly, and held away with a soft strap. The distal peroneal retinacula may have to be partially released. A small distractor is quite useful for a complete assessment of the joint and for correcting the length of the lateral column. The small Steinmann pins are placed into the anterior process of the calcaneus and the tuberosity of the fifth metatarsal or the distal aspect of the cuboid.[1]

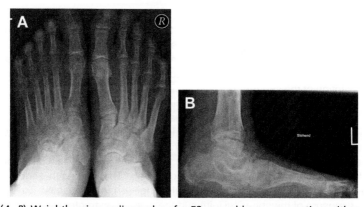

Fig. 9. (*A, B*) Weightbearing radiographs of a 52-year-old man presenting with a complex malunion of the foot 11 months after a transnavicular, transcuboidal, and transcalcaneal Chopart fracture-dislocation (type III deformity). Note abduction of the forefoot, caused by a collapse of the lateral column, with subsequent development of a posttraumatic flatfoot.

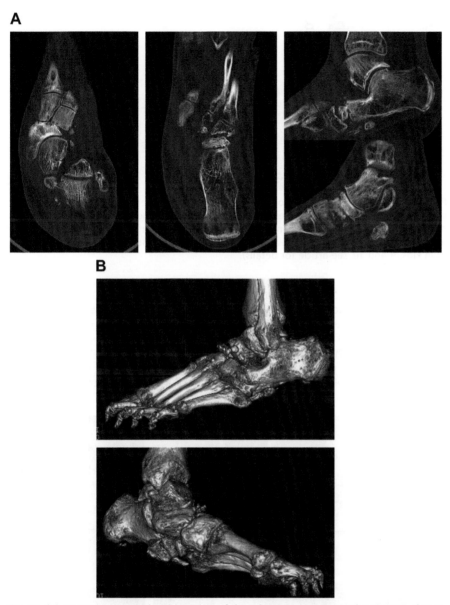

Fig. 10. (*A*) CT scanning reveals subluxation of the talonavicular joint without signs of post-traumatic arthritis, whereas the calcaneocuboid and naviculocuneiform display malunion and arthritis. (*B*) 3-dimensional reconstructions reveals the outline of the deformity (same patient as in **Fig. 9**, see article for details).

After clearing the joints from debris and adhesions, the joint cartilage can be probed and inspected directly and the definitive decision of secondary reconstruction versus corrective fusion is made at that time. In the following, the principles of joint-preserving correction will be demonstrated along with 3 characteristic case examples.

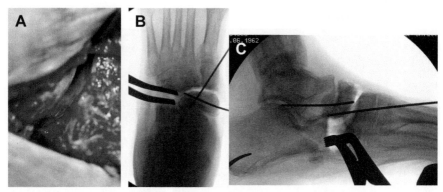

Fig. 11. (*A*) Intraoperative aspect of the talonavicular joint after distraction showing intact cartilage. (*B, C*) Fluoroscopic images showing realignment of the foot with reduction of the navicular medially and distraction of the cuboid laterally. Internal fixation was finally achieved with cervical plates, screws, and bone grafting to the lateral side (same patient as in **Figs. 9** and **10**, see article for details).

Correction of a Type I Deformity

Figs. 2–6 show anatomic reconstruction of a type I deformity in a 59-year-old man presenting with a painful malunion of the cuboid 5 months after an overlooked malunited transcuboidal Chopart fracture-dislocation. The radiographs demonstrate a double contour at the calcaneocuboid joint (see **Fig. 2**) resulting from the typical nutcracker fracture mechanism.[16] CT analysis reveals that the joint surface is impressed as a whole. Because the lateral wall of the cuboid is still in place and

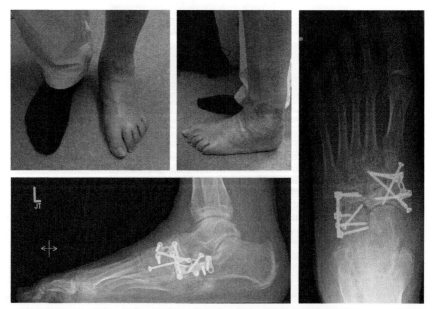

Fig. 12. Standing radiographs and clinical aspect 4 months after correction showing anatomic realignment, uneventful scars, and solid fusion (same patient as in **Figs. 9–11**, see article for details).

the joint impressed medially there is a slight paradoxic adduction of the midfoot (see **Fig. 3**). Intraoperatively, a complete cartilage cover is seen over the impressed joint surface of the cuboid and the corresponding facet of the calcaneus (see **Fig. 4**A). The lateral wall is resected and preserved, then a horizontal osteotomy was carried out parallel to the depressed joint surface (see **Fig. 4**B). The proximal portion carrying the joint surface is then elevated using the calcaneus as a template (see **Fig. 4**C). A lateral distractor is placed between the anterior calcaneal process and the distal portion of the cuboid to maintain the correct length. The resected lateral wall of the cuboid is used as a bone graft (see **Fig. 4**D). Fixation is achieved with an interlocking anatomic cuboid plate. Weightbearing radiographs at 1 year show anatomic alignment. The cuboid has solidly healed with minimal lateral osteophyte formation (see **Fig. 5**). The patient has no pain during the activities of daily living. Clinical images show uneventful scars and near-normal range of motion in the horizontal and sagittal plane (see **Fig. 6**).

Correction of a Type II Deformity

Figs. 7 and **8** show anatomic reconstruction of a navicular nonunion in a 24-year-old man presenting 2 years after a traffic accident with multiple injuries. Nonunion of the plantar aspect of the navicular is detected in plain radiographs and the exact extent is confirmed with CT scanning (see **Fig. 7**). After placement of a joint distractor the whole surface of the talar head and navicular can be assessed and reveal a full cartilage cover (see **Fig. 8**A). Treatment consisted of careful debridement, bone grafting, and screw fixation of the navicular (see **Fig. 8**B). At 3 months, the navicular has solidly healed (see **Fig. 8**C).

Correction of a Type III Deformity

Figs. 9–12 shows correction of a type III deformity in a 52-year-old man presenting with a complex malunion 11 months after K-wire fixation of a transnavicular, transcuboidal, and transcalcaneal Chopart fracture-dislocation. The patient is unable to walk without crutches and takes daily pain medications. Standing radiographs demonstrate a severe abduction of the forefoot, caused by a collapse of the lateral column, with subsequent development of a posttraumatic flatfoot (see **Fig. 9**). CT scanning reveals a defect in the cuboid involving the calcaneocuboid joint while the talonavicular joint is subluxed but without step-offs or signs of posttraumatic arthritis (see **Fig. 10**). Instead, the malunion causing talonavicular dislocation is at the level of the naviculocuneiform joints that show manifest arthritic changes. Intraoperative exposure of the talonavicular joint shows a complete cartilage cover over the talar head and navicular with first-degree to second-degree chondromalacia (see **Fig. 11**A). Correction of the deformity was achieved by step-wise mobilization and reduction of the navicular from medial using 2 K-wires as joysticks and distraction of the lateral side using a laminar spreader (see **Fig. 11**B). The length of the lateral column was restored by corrective fusion of the calcaneocuboid joint with bone grafting from the iliac crest. The medial column was stabilized by fusion of the naviculocuneiform joints while the talonavicular joint could be preserved. Four months after the correction, the fusions are fully consolidated. Standing radiographs and clinical images show a plantigrade foot with axial realignment (see **Fig. 12**).

IMMEDIATE POSTOPERATIVE CARE AND REHABILITATION

The operated foot is put in a splint or split below-knee cast. If no temporary joint transfixation was performed, physical therapy with active and passive range-of-motion exercises starts on the second postoperative day. Any suction drain is removed at that time. At 5 to 7 days, a walking cast, special boot, or walker is fitted and patients are mobilized with partial weightbearing of about 20 kg.

After osteotomy with bone grafting, partial weightbearing with 20 kg is maintained for 10 to 12 weeks postoperatively in the lower-leg cast or boot.

Physical therapy is continued without loading and intensified when full weightbearing is allowed after radiologic confirmation of bone healing. It then includes gait training, muscle strengthening, and proprioceptive exercises to achieve a near physiologic gait pattern. Removal of implants is only advised if a protrusion is felt by the patient or in combination with other procedures. Surgical revision may also be indicated in case of restricted motion, nonunion of the osteotomy, AVN, or progressive arthritis requiring fusion.[19,21,22]

CLINICAL RESULTS FROM THE LITERATURE

The mainstay of salvage procedures after Chopart joint malunion is corrective arthrodesis of the affected joints to restore alignment and stability of the foot. Several investigators have described partial functional rehabilitation and substantial reduction of pain after talonavicular, calcaneocuboidal, double or triple fusion for posttraumatic arthritis, malunion, nonunion, or AVN.[10,20,21,23–26] Until recently, joint-sparing corrections of malunited Chopart joint injuries have only been reported anecdotally.[7] In 2010, Rammelt and colleagues[1] first reported on a small series of 8 subjects who were treated with secondary anatomic reconstruction of malunion and nonunion at the Chopart joint. At 2 years follow-up, all subjects but 1 were satisfied with the result and foot functions had improved substantially.

More recently, a follow-up of this series was reported.[22] It included 16 subjects with joint-preserving corrections for malunion and nonunion at the Chopart joint: 6 at the navicular, 3 at the talar head, 3 at the anterior calcaneal process, 2 at the cuboid, and 2 with combined malunion. Mean subject age was 32 years (range 14–69 years). Subjects presented at an average of 7 months (range 1.5–15 months) after the initial injury. There were 7 cases of type I and 8 cases of type II deformities. One patient with a type IV deformity was treated with corrective talonavicular fusion and a lengthening osteotomy of the cuboid, thus saving the calcaneocuboid joint. The average American Orthopaedic Foot and Ankle Society (AOFAS) score significantly increased from 37 preoperatively to 77 at final follow-up in 12 subjects at an average of 2 years after correction. Two female subjects, ages 50 and 67, developed AVN of the navicular and required talonavicular fusion and 1 subject with a nonunion of the anterior calcaneal process needed a second revision surgery for obtaining union. The best results were achieved in young subjects with higher potential bone and joint remodeling even after long-standing joint displacement. It was concluded that joint-sparing osteotomies may be performed even more generously in adolescents.[22]

SUMMARY

The main goal when treating malunion and nonunion at the Chopart joint is axial realignment of the midfoot to the hindfoot and restoration of the physiologic relationship of the lateral and medial columns of the foot. In carefully selected cases, joint-preserving osteotomies are generally possible at all 4 bony components of the Chopart joint to restore near-normal foot function. Priority should be given to the anatomic reconstruction of the talonavicular joint because, as part of the coxa pedis, it is essential for global foot function. However, patients must be counseled about the risk of progressive arthritis or osteonecrosis necessitating late fusion. In patients with symptomatic posttraumatic arthritis, extensile AVN, ongoing infection, severe comorbidities, or poor compliance, arthrodesis with realignment and bone grafting remains the treatment of choice.

REFERENCES

1. Rammelt S, Zwipp H, Schneiders W, et al. Anatomical reconstruction after malunited Chopart joint injuries. Eur J Trauma Emerg Med 2010;36:196–205.
2. Zwipp H, Rammelt S. Tscherne Unfallchirurgie: Fuß. Berlin; Heidelberg (Germany); New York: Springer-Verlag; 2014.
3. van Dorp KB, de Vries MR, van der Elst M, et al. Chopart joint injury: a study of outcome and morbidity. J Foot Ankle Surg 2010;49(6):541–5.
4. Benirschke SK, Meinberg E, Anderson SA, et al. Fractures and dislocations of the midfoot: Lisfranc and Chopart injuries. J Bone Joint Surg Am 2012;94-A(14): 1325–37.
5. Main BJ, Jowett RL. Injuries of the midtarsal joint. J Bone Joint Surg Br 1975;57-B: 89–97.
6. Kotter A, Wieberneit J, Braun W, et al. The Chopart dislocation. A frequently underestimated injury and its sequelae. A clinical study. Unfallchirurg 1997;100:737–41.
7. Rammelt S, Grass R, Schikore H, et al. Verletzungen des Chopart-Gelenks. Unfallchirurg 2002;105(4):371–85.
8. Richter M, Thermann H, Huefner T, et al. Chopart joint fracture-dislocation: initial open reduction provides better outcome than closed reduction. Foot Ankle Int 2004;25:340–8.
9. Rammelt S, Thielemann F, Zwipp H. Reconstruction of malunited Chopart fracture-dislocations. FussSprungg 2009;7:105–17.
10. Zwipp H, Rammelt S. Posttraumatic deformity correction at the foot. Zentralbl Chir 2003;128:218–26.
11. Klaue K. Chopart fractures. Injury 2004;35(Suppl 2):SB64–70.
12. Manter JT. Movements of the subtalar and transverse tarsal joints. Anat Rec 1941; 80:397–410.
13. Astion DJ, Deland JT, Otis JC, et al. Motion of the hindfoot after simulated arthrodesis. J Bone Joint Surg Am 1997;79:241–6.
14. Wülker N, Stukenborg C, Savory KM, et al. Hindfoot motion after isolated and combined arthrodeses: measurements in anatomic specimens. Foot Ankle Int 2000;21:921–7.
15. Deland JT, Otis JC, Lee KT, et al. Lateral column lengthening with calcaneocuboid fusion: range of motion in the triple joint complex. Foot Ankle Int 1995;16:729–33.
16. Hermel MB, Gershon-Cohen J. The nutcracker fracture of the cuboid by indirect violence. Radiology 1953;60:850–3.
17. Zwipp H. Chirurgie des Fußes. Wien (Austria); New York: Springer-Verlag; 1994.
18. Suckel A, Müller O, Langenstein P, et al. Chopart's joint load during gait. In vitro study of 10 cadaver specimen in a dynamic model. Gait Posture 2008;27:216–22.
19. Rammelt S. Chopart and Lisfranc joint injuries. In: Bentley G, editor. European surgical orthopaedics and traumatology. The EFORT textbook. Berlin; Heidelberg (Germany); New York: Springer; 2014. p. 3835–57.
20. Laing AJ, Sangeorzan BJ. Post traumatic reconstruction of the foot and ankle—principles of correction. FussSprungg 2009;7:70–7.
21. Adelaar RS. Complications of forefoot and midfoot fractures. Clin Orthop Relat Res 2001;391:26–32.

22. Rammelt S, Zwipp H. Joint-preserving correction of Chopart joint malunions. Unfallchirurg 2014;117:785–90.
23. Rammelt S, Marti RK, Zwipp H. Arthrodesis of the talonavicular joint. Orthopade 2006;35:428–34.
24. Penner MJ. Late reconstruction after navicular fracture. Foot Ankle Clin 2006; 11(1):105–19, ix.
25. Smith RW, Shen W, Dewitt S, et al. Triple arthrodesis in adults with non-paralytic disease. A minimum ten-year follow-up study. J Bone Joint Surg Am 2004;86-A: 2707–13.
26. Kettunen J, Kroger H. Surgical treatment of ankle and foot fractures in the elderly. Osteoporos Int 2005;16(suppl 2):S103–6.

Joint-sparing Corrections in Malunited Lisfranc Joint Injuries

Caio Nery, MD, PhD[a,b,]*, Fernando Raduan, MD[a,b], Daniel Baumfeld, MD[c,d]

KEYWORDS

- Lisfranc malunion • Neoligamentplasty • Midfoot deformity

KEY POINTS

- An asymmetric midfoot with incongruent joints changes the normal foot shape leading to shoe wearing problems and gait disorders.
- Significant deformities cannot be corrected with ligamentplasty or endobutton stabilization; the latter should be reserved for subtle instabilities with ligamentous disruption and without arthritic changes.
- Neoligamentoplasty allows for reconstruction of 3 types of ligamentous disruption and the endobutton technique primarily reconstructs the Lisfranc ligament.
- Dorsal bridging plates can provide rigid fixation and allow for correction of greater deformities of the midfoot but require a large exposure of the tarsometatarsal joints.
- It is preferable to have an incomplete correction than to close the incision under tension.

INTRODUCTION

Ligament injuries and fracture–dislocations of the intercuneiform and tarsometatarsal (TMT) joints (Lisfranc) are relatively uncommon.[1,2] The seemingly low incidence is probably owing to misdiagnosed or overlooked injuries (20% and 40%, respectively) treated as foot sprains.[3,4] The subtle injuries represent a major source of initially missed or misinterpreted lesions, which may lead to chronic pain and functional loss owing to deformity, residual ligamentous instability, or arthritis.[5,6] It is generally accepted that displaced or unstable Lisfranc injuries are treated with anatomic reduction and stabilization of the Lisfranc joints to achieve good outcomes and avoid deleterious sequelae. If overlooked or not treated correctly, TMT fracture–dislocations frequently result in painful malunion and impaired function.

The authors have nothing to disclose.

[a] Albert Einstein Hospital, Foot and Ankle Clinic, Hospital Israelita Albert Einstein, Avenue Albert Einstein, 627, Bloco A1 - 3o andar, sala 317, Morumbi, São Paulo, Brazil; [b] UNIFESP - Federal University of São Paulo - Foot and Ankle Surgery, São Paulo, Brazil; [c] Hospital Felicio Rocho, Belo Horizonte, Minas Gerais, Brazil; [d] UFMG - Federal University of Minas Gerais - Foot and Ankle Surgery, Minas Gerais, Brazil
* Corresponding author.
E-mail address: caioneryprof@gmail.com

Inveterate Lisfranc fractures or dislocations are defined as being more than 6 to 12 weeks old and these injuries can be anatomically reconstructed only in rare cases.[7] A key issue in determining whether a reconstruction should be performed is whether the joint is viable and without degeneration.

PATIENT ASSESSMENT

Disability assessment and treatment are difficult because of the presence of different symptoms, which cause overlapping syndromes. Patients complain of pain, walking limitations, and necessity to change their lifestyle. A careful and detailed clinical assessment followed by an extensive radiologic investigation will usually reveal 1 or more of the following problems.

LISFRANC JOINT MALALIGNMENT

Lisfranc joint malalignment can occur in multiple planes and depends on the type of primary injury. Most commonly, planus or planovalgus deformities associated with forefoot abduction are seen but cavus deformity with forefoot adduction may also be encountered[8–10] (**Fig. 1**).

Zwipp[7,11] staged a Lisfranc joint malposition with or without osteoarthritis:

1. Lisfranc ligament instability without osteoarthritis (**Fig. 2**).
2. Medial (cuneiform I-III/metatarsal I-III) Lisfranc osteoarthritis and/or malposition.
3. Lateral (cuboid/metatarsal IV-V) Lisfranc osteoarthritis and/or malposition.
4. Lisfranc osteoarthritis medially and laterally in pes planovalgus with abduction.
5. Lisfranc osteoarthritis medially and laterally with pes cavovarus.

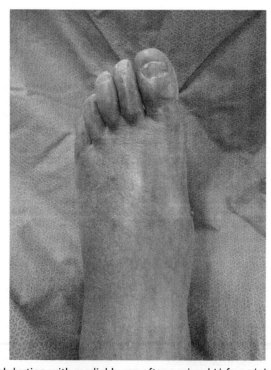

Fig. 1. Forefoot abduction with medial bump after a missed Lisfranc injury.

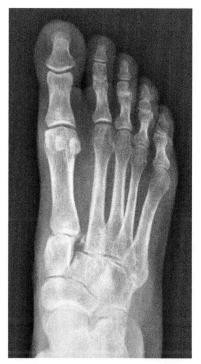

Fig. 2. Lisfranc ligament instability demonstrated with a standing anteroposterior radiograph.

Tarsometatarsal Bossing and Metatarsalgia

Tenderness and bossing may exist over the TMT, naviculocuneiform, or calcaneocuboid joints. An asymmetric midfoot with incongruent joints changes the normal foot shape, leading to shoe wearing problems and gait disorders, usually owing to decreased push-off strength[12] (**Fig. 3**). Inspection and verification of painful calluses under the metatarsal heads with transfer metatarsalgia results in altered medial arch height during standing; hyperkeratosis under the navicular in abduction-type deformities may also be present.[13,14]

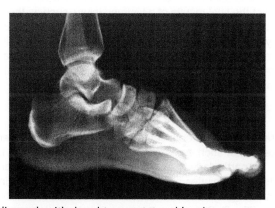

Fig. 3. Lateral radiograph with dorsal tarsometatarsal bossing.

PREOPERATIVE IMAGING

Anteroposterior (AP) and lateral weight-bearing radiographs of both feet and a non–weight-bearing 45° oblique view permit an assessment of alignment and foot axis. The normal Lisfranc joint alignment should follow the criteria below[3] (**Fig. 4**):

1. The shaft of the first metatarsal projects in line with the longitudinal axis of the medial cuneiform on the AP view;
2. The talus first metatarsal axis should be straight in both the AP and lateral projections;
3. The distance between the bases of the first and second metatarsal should not exceed 3 mm on AP radiographs;
4. The medial contour of the second metatarsal basis should be in line with the medial edge of the intermediate cuneiform also on AP view;
5. The medial contour of the fourth metatarsal should be in line with the medial edge of the cuboid bone on the 45° oblique projection;
6. There should not be any visible vertical deviation of the metatarsal bases with regard to the cuneiforms on the lateral projection; and
7. Alignment view of the fifth metatarsal basis inferiorly to the medial cuneiform in standing lateral radiographs; in chronic ligamentous instability of the first ray, the inferior border of the medial cuneiform projects below the base of the fifth metatarsal.

AP abduction stress radiographs confirm the diagnosis in selected cases of suspected latent instability.[5] Computed tomography scan may be useful for the preoperative analysis of posttraumatic osteoarthritis, osseous defects, and subtle deformities[15,16] (**Fig. 5**). A MRI scan may only be helpful in the diagnosis of acute, purely ligamentous injuries and assessment of the extent of osteonecrosis and differential diagnosis of acute Charcot feet.[3,17]

Decision Making

The best results in the treatment of TMT injuries are achieved with stable anatomic reduction.[18,19] Surgery should be delayed until edema has decreased, minimizing wound complications.[20] The literature is sparse with respect to the best timing for open reduction and internal fixation (ORIF) of Lisfranc injuries when they are no longer acute. Kuo and associates[21] found no difference in the outcome scores between acute and delayed (>6 weeks; 3 patients) ORIF of Lisfranc injuries. Patients with purely ligamentous injuries had poorer outcomes. The literature also listed other features that can negatively affect the final results of a Lisfranc injury, such as the lack of anatomic reduction, significant fracture comminution, and when the diagnosis was missed or significantly delayed.[2,20,22–24] The incidence of posttraumatic arthritis after TMT injuries ranges from 0% to 58%.[25] One can decide between joint-sparing procedures or arthrodesis considering the amount of joint arthritis, time of primary injury, midfoot deformity, and patient cooperation.

CONSERVATIVE TREATMENT OF LISFRANC MALUNION

Patients should be warned that conservative treatment will not correct the deformity and the main objective of such surgery is pain relief. Immobilization in a cast or cam walker boot may be particularly helpful in decreasing pain and promoting ligament healing in patients whose injuries are only a few weeks old. A rigid insole with a thin carbon fiber lamina along with a rocker bottom shoe may aid ambulation without overloading the midfoot (**Fig. 6**). Specific custom-made orthosis (University of California or

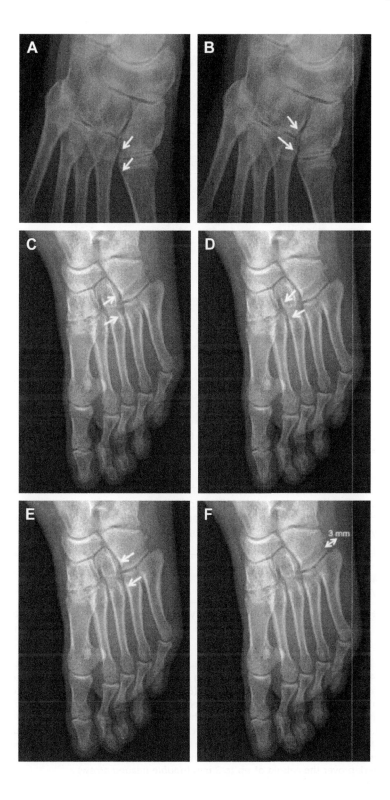

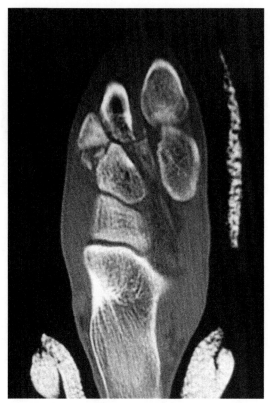

Fig. 5. Computed tomography scan showing fragmentation from the base of the second metatarsal.

Arizona brace) can support the arch, accommodate fixed deformity, limit the subluxation owing to ligamentous instability, and decrease painful motion of arthritic joints.[5,20] Glucosamine/chondroitin sulfate and nonsteroidal antiinflammatory medication may be prescribed for pain relief. Patients must either limit or avoid sports activities.

SURGICAL TREATMENT
Patient Warning

This type of treatment involves major surgery and the patient must understand that, if it fails, arthrodesis remains an option. The possibility of wound breakdown, deep

Fig. 4. (*A*) Anteroposterior (AP) view showing alignment of the lateral cortex of the medial cuneiform and the first metatarsal (*arrows*). (*B*) AP view showing alignment of the medial cortex of the middle cuneiform and the second metatarsal (*arrows*). (*C*) Oblique view showing alignment of the lateral cortex of the lateral cuneiform and the third metatarsal (*arrows*). (*D*) Oblique view showing alignment of the medial cortex of the lateral cuneiform and the third metatarsal (*arrows*). (*E*) Oblique view showing alignment of the medial cortex of the cuboid and the fourth metatarsal (*arrows*). (*F*) Oblique view showing the fifth metatarsal overlap over the cuboid of up to 3 mm (*double headed arrow*).

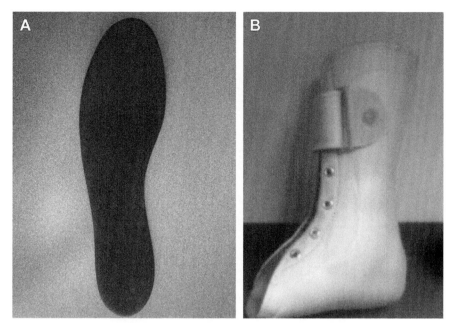

Fig. 6. (*A*) Rigid insole. (*B*) Custom made orthesis.

surgical site infection, and painful scarring of the dorsum of the foot should be discussed as well. The reconstruction results are reasonable but by no means perfect.[20,26] The vascular status of the foot must be excellent, and the patient should stop smoking.

Patient Position and Incision

The principles of this treatment are the same as those for acute Lisfranc injuries.[27] The presence of interposed scar tissue between the metatarsal bones usually imposes an open reduction with the patient in the supine position under regional anesthesia and sedation, with the ankle and foot being placed in a neutral position. We recommend a thigh pneumatic tourniquet to allow proper visualization of the injured joints. An approach can be made through 1 or 2 dorsal longitudinal incisions, depending on the extent of pathology. The first incision is made over the second TMT joint or between the first and second TMT joints. The first TMT joint may be exposed medially to the extensor hallucis longus tendon, avoiding injury to the dorsal medial cutaneous branch of the superficial peroneal nerve. It can also be exposed through the interval between the extensor hallucis longus and extensor hallucis brevis, which allows access to the medial–intermediate intercuneiform joint, medial cuneiform–second metatarsal articulation, and Lisfranc ligament. Care must be taken with the dorsalis pedis artery and deep peroneal nerve. If required, the incision can be extended proximally to access the naviculocuneiform joint. If the lateral TMT joints do not correct after reduction of the medial TMT joints, a second longitudinal incision is made in line with the fourth TMT joint or the interval between the third and fourth TMT joints.[10] It is important to preserve the superficial peroneal nerve branches (**Fig. 7**).

Alternatively, the region of the intercuneiforms and TMT joints can be exposed through a transverse dorsal incision, which allows an excellent visualization of all

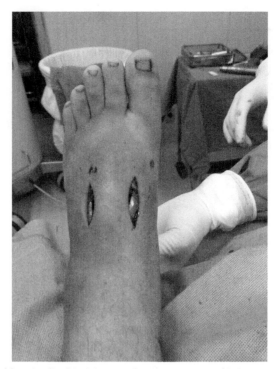

Fig. 7. Two dorsal longitudinal incisions to the tarsometatarsal joints.

TMT joints.[28] The transverse incision has the advantage of clearly expose the damaged structures and local deformities, greatly helping to reduce deviations and carrying out bone tunnels; however, it offers substantial risk to the dorsal nerve vascular bundle and should be performed with extreme caution.

It is important to identify all torn structures and remove all ligament remnants, particularly in the interosseous layer, facilitating anatomic reduction and preventing persistent pain. The results of this meticulous revision and debridement are the reestablishment of a normal intercuneiform and TMT joint relationship.

SURGICAL NEOLIGAMENTPLASTY

This technique is a safe and viable alternative to the classic procedures in the treatment of acute or late subtle intercuneiform and TMT joint lesions.[29] The concept is to reconstruct the stabilizing ligaments of the Lisfranc joint with a tendon graft through bone tunnels. Regarding the strength of ligamentous reconstruction, some authors have demonstrated that tendon fixation can provide similar stability to screw fixation in Lisfranc ligamentous injury.[30] It is advised that a significant number of deformities cannot be corrected with this reconstruction technique and it should be reserved for subtle instability after purely ligamentous disruption.

TECHNIQUE
Bone Tunnels

According to the anatomic orientation of the original ligaments, there are 3 main tunnels that have to be made before reconstructing the original ligament anatomy (**Fig. 8**).

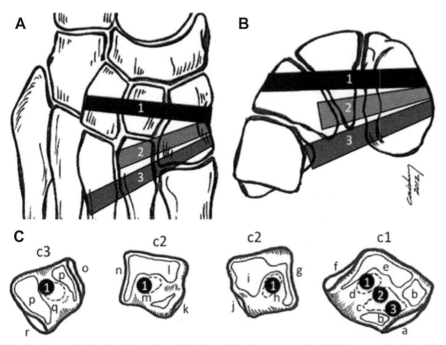

Fig. 8. Anatomic landmarks and positioning of the bone tunnels. (*A*) Transversal plane. (*B*) Coronal plane. (*C*) Cuneiform bones: C1a-f, lateral surface of the first cuneiform; C2g-j, medial surface of the second cuneiform; C2k-n, lateral surface of the second cuneiform; C3o-r, medial surface of the third cuneiform. 1, drill hole for the first tunnel; 2, drill hole for the second tunnel; 3, drill hole for the third tunnel; a, articular surface for the first metatarsal; b, articular surface for the second metatarsal; c, insertional zone of the Lisfranc ligament; d, Insertional zone of intercuneiform C1 to C2 ligament; e, articular surface to the second cuneiform; f, articular surface to the navicular bone; g, articular surface to the navicular bone; h, insertional zone of intercuneiform C1 to C2 ligament; i, articular surface to the first cuneiform; j, articular surface to the second metatarsal; k, articular surface to the second metatarsal; l, articular surface to the third cuneiform; m, insertional zone of intercuneiform C2 to C3 ligament; n, articular surface to the navicular bone; o, articular surface to the navicular bone; p, articular surface to the second cuneiform; q, insertional zone of intercuneiform C2 to C3 ligament; r, articular surface to the third metatarsal. (*From* Nery C, Ressio C, Alloza JFM. Subtle Lisfranc joint ligament lesions: surgical neoligamentplasty technique. Foot Ankle Clin N Am 2012;17:414; with permission.)

- After an extensive and careful reduction of each of the identified joint asymmetries, the temporary stabilization of the region was achieved with K-wires and bone clamps. Then the bone tunnels are drilled, passed, and the graft fixed.
- The first transverse tunnel (recreates the cuneiform interosseous ligaments) runs from the deep point of the first cuneiforms medial aspect depression to the midpoint of the third cuneiform dorsolateral border. When correctly oriented, this tunnel crosses the geometric center of the first cuneiform, the distal one-half of the second cuneiform, and the geometric center of the third cuneiform, preserving all articular surfaces of these 3 bones.
- The second oblique tunnel (reproduces Lisfranc's ligament) runs from the medial aspect of the first cuneiform to the proximal metaphysis of the second

metatarsal. When correctly oriented, this tunnel crosses the contact region between the first cuneiform and the base of the second metatarsal.
- The third plantar tunnel (reproduces the deep plantar ligaments) is the most anterior tunnel and runs obliquely from the first cuneiform to the base of the third metatarsal.

It is not always necessary to use all of the 3 tunnels described. To achieve the best and most stable correction possible, the surgeon must decide which tunnels are needed and the best sequence to drive the harvested tendon into the tunnels.

GRAFT

This technique is recommended for the third extensor digitorum longus, reinforced by a #2 fiber-wire (Arthrex, Naples, FL) suture as a preferred graft. Alternatively, a hamstring muscle or an allograft can be used (**Fig. 9**). Care must be taken when harvesting the extensor digitorum longus because the graft must be at least 9 cm long to complete the procedure as described.

Joint Stabilization

The neoligament graft is guided through the tunnel with the help of a tendon passer, and the correct tension is applied to the ends of the sutures with a bone reduction forceps in place to ensure the stability and flexibility of the joints.

- Before considering the completion of the procedure, the bone forceps are removed and a supination–pronation maneuver is repeated to check the efficiency and accuracy of the construct.

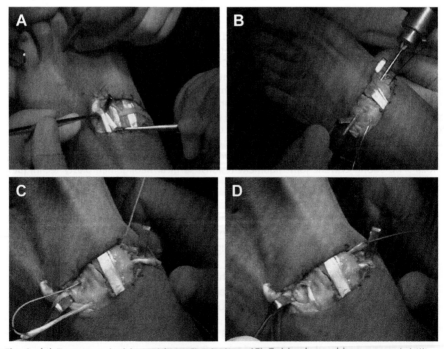

Fig. 9. (*A*) Transverse incision with graft selection. (*B*) Guidewire and bone tunnel drilling. (*C*) Graft passed medial to lateral. (*D*) U-shaped graft passed medial to lateral and then lateral to medial.

- The knots should be hidden between the bones, in the interosseous musculature or inside the tunnels.
- A biotenodesis screw can be used for bone/tendon fixation

Postoperative Considerations

The incision is closed in the usual manner and a short neutral lower leg splint is used for 3 weeks. The skin sutures are removed on postoperative day 21. The patient must adhere to an 8-week non–weight-bearing period followed by a 3-month rehabilitation program that consists of progressive weight-bearing, gait training, range of motion exercised (lower limb joints), muscle strengthening (thigh, leg and foot), proprioception, and balance.

NONRIGID (ENDOBUTTON) STABILIZATION

The concept of nonrigid fixation has been previously explored using biological substitutes such as the extensor tendons and hamstring tendons.[21,31] The fixation using the endobutton (TightRope Arthrex) technique avoids donor site morbidity. The advantages of nonrigid fixation include avoiding screw breakage and the need for implant removal.[32] Rigid fixation locks the joints leading to impairment of foot kinematics functioning as an arthrodesis. This technique follows the same indications as the neoligamentoplasty and should be used in injuries with subtle instability and no gross deformity. The differences in these 2 techniques are: (1) neoligamentoplasty allows reconstruction of 3 different ligamentous disruption patterns (2) endo-button technique primarily reconstructs an isolated chronic Lisfranc ligament instability.

TECHNIQUE

- The second metatarsal base must be accurately reduced to the intercuneiform "keystone" recess, using large bone reduction forceps (**Fig. 10**).
- Satisfactory reduction is confirmed by means of intraoperative fluoroscopy.
- Insertion of a guide wire in the direction of the injured ligament, from the medial cuneiform through the base of the second metatarsal is required (see **Fig. 10**A).
- A 2.7-mm cannulated drill is used to allow insertion of the device.
- The device is inserted percutaneously under fluoroscopic guidance.
- The TightRope device is pulled through the tunnel. The oblong button has to align easily along the lateral second metatarsal cortex, which is checked with fluoroscopy (see **Fig. 10**B).
- The wires are pulled simultaneously to tighten the system and the round button should lie snugly over the medial cuneiform wall. To ensure stability, the medial and lateral buttons must be placed on the bone itself with no soft tissue or tendon interpositions (see **Fig. 10**C).
- After tightening the device, the bone clamp is released (see **Fig. 10**D).
- At the end of the operation, the foot is kept in a non–weight-bearing cast for 3 weeks. Afterward, the cast is removed and physical therapy initiated. Full weight bearing is allowed after 6 weeks.

Dorsal Plating Without Transarticular Screws

The concept of dorsal plate fixation instead of transarticular screws in reconstructing the Lisfranc joint is to avoid further damage to the joints already traumatized by the initial injury or chronic malposition.[33,34] Dorsal plates can provide rigid fixation without

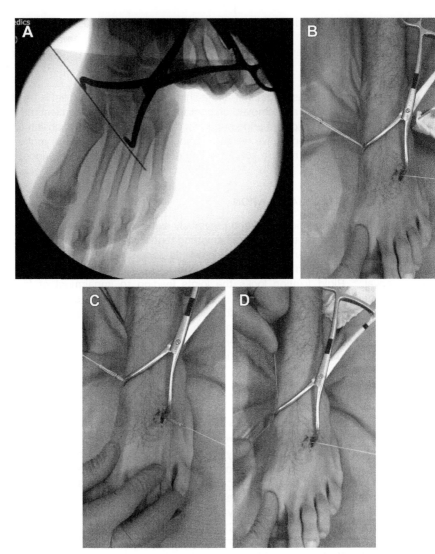

Fig. 10. (*A*) Positioning of the reduction forceps. (*B*) The construct is passed through the bone tunnel. (*C*) Tighten the endo-button system. (*D*) Suture ends cut and reduction clamp released.

further damage to the articular surface but this needs a large exposition of the TMT joint.[35] This technique is commonly used for the medial rays (first, second, and third) and allows for correction of greater deformities of the midfoot.[34] The plates work as a bridge between the metatarsals and the cuneiforms.

TECHNIQUE
Reduction

- The first step is to reduce the unstable joints, starting with the first or second TMT joint.[33–35] Reduction is maintained with a pointed reduction forceps followed by a K-wire. Additional K-wires are placed across the Lisfranc joint and from the base of the second metatarsal into the second cuneiform.

- In cases of displacement of the third TMT joint, a second approach is made between the third and fourth metatarsals.

Fixation

- After reduction, small fragment plates (2.4–2.7 mm) are applied dorsally across the first and/or second and/or third TMT joints, according to what is required, without compression or crossing screws (**Fig. 11**).
- The plates should be designed to fit 3 screws in the cuneiform and first metatarsal. Additional plates across the second and third metatarsals should also be applied, depending on the amount of bony deformity and instability.
- It is important not only to preserve the original anatomic first metatarsal flexion and adduction, but also the relationship between the second and third metatarsal with the respective cuneiforms.
- The edges of the reduced joints must match both visually and under fluoroscopy using AP, oblique and lateral views as described.
- If there is gross instability between the first and the second metatarsal, a single screw between the first cuneiform and second metatarsal, and between the first and second cuneiform should be inserted. This eliminates residual intercolumn instability.

Postoperative Care

- A bellow-knee non–weight-bearing boot is used for 8 weeks.
- Foot and ankle range of motion exercises are initiated at 3 weeks.
- At 2 months, patients are allowed to increase weight bearing as tolerated.
- Plates and screws are routinely removed during the fourth month and patients are permitted to fully bear weight on the limb.

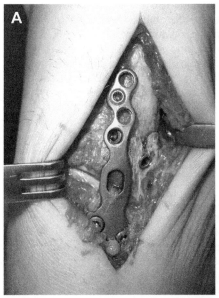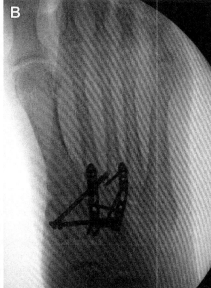

Fig. 11. (*A*) First tarsometatarsal (TMT) joint bridge plate. (*B*) Second and third TMT joint bridge plates.

CLINICAL RESULTS IN THE LITERATURE

Generally, it is recommended that surgery for Lisfranc fractures and dislocations should be performed within 6 weeks of the injury,[36,37] but Chiodo and Myerson[38] have reduced TMT joint dislocations successfully with ORIF at 1 year after injury. They stated that the success of such a late reduction depends on the extent of articular incongruity and cannot be accomplished in the presence of a malunited fracture. In their case series of 9 patients, 2 with late Lisfranc injuries, Aitken and Poulsen[39] found good functional results, despite persistent dislocations. Trevino and Kodros[37] stated that, although good results have been obtained as late as 6 weeks after injury, the success of surgery after 6 weeks is diminished by multiple factors, including the need for extensive soft tissue dissection, destruction of articular surface because of malposition, and suboptimal stabilization of the Lisfranc ligament. In another report, 13 patients who underwent ORIF more than 6 weeks (average 31.8 weeks) after Lisfranc joint injury were compared with 42 patients who underwent surgery within weeks of injury at an average follow-up period of 49.4 months. The group that had delayed diagnosis, all of whom had sustained pure ligamentous injuries without fractures, had a lower postoperative American Orthopedic Foot and Ankle Society midfoot score (64 vs 73.5) and a higher rate of subsequent midfoot arthrodesis (23% vs 9.5%).[20]

Other studies have shown worse outcomes after delayed treatment with arthrodesis compared with primary ORIF.[10] Nery and colleagues[29] reported treatment of 20 patients with ligamentous instability diagnosed between 1 week and 36 months (average 9 months) after injury with delayed reconstruction of the Lisfranc ligament. Poor results were observed in 3 patients and it was related to the time elapsed (20 months) between the trauma and diagnosis. Although it may seem natural that the delay in diagnosis may be responsible for generating worse results, we do not have objective data that can demonstrate the ideal time to define prognosis. The presence of old, displaced fragments in the region could also negatively affect the results.[29]

Few other reports exist on neoligamentoplasty for Lisfranc joint instability in young, active patients. Hirano and colleagues[40] used the gracilis tendon as a graft in a 15-year-old male patient with an acute Lisfranc ligament disruption and fractures of the second to fourth metatarsal bases. The authors report a full functional rehabilitation without residual complaints after 1 year. Zwipp and Rammelt[11] described 4 cases of reconstruction of the chronically unstable Lisfranc ligament with either half of the extensor hallucis longus or the whole extensor hallucis brevis tendon passed through V-shaped bone tunnels at the medial cuneiform and the second metatarsal base. Temporary joint transfixation was achieved with screws and K-wires for 8 weeks. All patients had a stable TMT joint up to 10 years with full return to preinjury activity, including 1 elite gymnast.

SUMMARY

Lisfranc fracture–dislocation is a serious and commonly missed injury. Frequent complications after a missed lesion include chronic edema, complex regional pain syndrome, forefoot abduction or adduction, planovalgus or cavovarus deformity, bony exostosis, and posttraumatic arthrosis. Anatomic reduction with the use of different types of internal fixation is necessary to reconstruct midfoot alignment and stability thus decreasing the morbidity of these injuries. The new surgical approaches for joint-sparing correction of missed Lisfranc injuries should be used with caution by an experienced surgeon. They allow full functional rehabilitation in young and active individuals.

REFERENCES

1. Hardcastle PH, Reschauer R, Kutscha-Lissberg E, et al. Injuries to the tarsome-tatarsal joint. Incidence, classification and treatment. J Bone Joint Surg Br 1982; 64:349–56.
2. Desmond EA, Chou LB. Current concepts review: Lisfranc injuries. Foot Ankle Int 2006;27:653–60.
3. Gupta RT, Wadhwa RP, Learch TJ, et al. Lisfranc injury: imaging findings for this important but often-missed diagnosis. Curr Probl Diagn Radiol 2008;37:115–26.
4. Saab M. Lisfranc fracture–dislocation: an easily overlooked injury in the emergency department. Eur J Emerg Med 2005;12:143–6.
5. Aronow MS. Treatment of the missed Lisfranc injury. Foot Ankle Clin 2006;11: 127–42.
6. Ly TV, Coetzee JC. Treatment of primarily ligamentous Lisfranc joint injuries: primary arthrodesis compared with open reduction and internal fixation. A prospective, randomized study. J Bone Joint Surg Am 2006;88:514–20.
7. Zwipp H. Reconstructions after inveterated fractures and dislocations of the foot. Orthopade 2014;43:1025–39.
8. Mittlmeier T, Beck M. Tarsometatarsal injuries–an often neglected entity. Ther Umsch 2004;61:459–65.
9. Zwipp H, Rammelt S, Holch M, et al. Lisfranc arthrodesis after malunited fracture healing. Unfallchirurg 1999;102:918–23.
10. Rammelt S, Schneiders W, Schikore H, et al. Primary open reduction and fixation compared with delayed corrective arthrodesis in the treatment of tarsometatarsal (Lisfranc) fracture dislocation. J Bone Joint Surg Br 2008;90:1499–506.
11. Zwipp H, Rammelt S. Anatomical reconstruction of chronically instable Lisfranc's ligaments. Unfallchirurg 2014;117:791–7.
12. Adelaar RS. Complications of forefoot and midfoot fractures. Clin Orthop Relat Res 2001;(391):26–32.
13. Tarczyńska M, Gawęda K, Dajewski Z, et al. Comparison of treatment results of acute and late injuries of the Lisfranc joint. Acta Ortop Bras 2013;21:344–3446.
14. Zgonis T, Burns P, Gehl R. Lisfranc arthrodesis. Clin Podiatr Med Surg 2004;21: 113–28, vi.
15. Loh SY, Soon JL, Verhoeven WJ. Tarsometatarsal joint injuries–review of clinical presentation and surgical treatment. Med J Malaysia 2005;60:71–5.
16. Sherief TI, Mucci B, Greiss M. Lisfranc injury: how frequently does it get missed? And how can we improve? Injury 2007;38:856–60.
17. Delfaut EM, Rosenberg ZS, Demondion X. Malalignment at the Lisfranc joint: MR features in asymptomatic patients and cadaveric specimens. Skeletal Radiol 2002;31:499–504.
18. Myerson M. The diagnosis and treatment of injuries to the Lisfranc joint complex. Orthop Clin North Am 1989;20:655–64.
19. Bandac RC, Botez P. Lisfranc midfoot dislocations: correlations between surgical treatment and functional outcomes. Rev Med Chir Soc Med Nat Iasi 2012;116: 834–9.
20. Philbin T, Rosenberg G, Sferra JJ. Complications of missed or untreated Lisfranc injuries. Foot Ankle Clin 2003;8:61–71.
21. Kuo RS, Tejwani NC, Digiovanni CW, et al. Outcome after open reduction and internal fixation of Lisfranc joint injuries. J Bone Joint Surg Am 2000;82:1609–18.
22. Coetzee JC. Making sense of Lisfranc injuries. Foot Ankle Clin 2008;13: 695–704, ix.

23. Crates JM, Barber FA, Sanders EJ. Subtle Lisfranc subluxation: results of operative and nonoperative treatment. J Foot Ankle Surg 2015;54(3):350–5.
24. Eleftheriou KI, Rosenfeld PF, Calder JD. Lisfranc injuries: an update. Knee Surg Sports Traumatol Arthrosc 2013;21:1434–46.
25. Watson TS, Shurnas PS, Denker J. Treatment of Lisfranc joint injury: current concepts. J Am Acad Orthop Surg 2010;18:718–28.
26. Teng AL, Pinzur MS, Lomasney L, et al. Functional outcome following anatomic restoration of tarsal-metatarsal fracture dislocation. Foot Ankle Int 2002;23:922–6.
27. van Rijn J, Dorleijn DM, Boetes B, et al. Missing the Lisfranc fracture: a case report and review of the literature. J Foot Ankle Surg 2012;51:270–4.
28. Vertullo CJ, Easley ME, Nunley JA. The transverse dorsal approach to the Lisfranc joint. Foot Ankle Int 2002;23:420–6.
29. Nery C, Réssio C, Marion Alloza JF. Neoligamentplasty for the treatment of subtle ligament lesions of the intercuneiform and tarsometatarsal joints. Tech Foot Ankle Surg 2010;9:92–9.
30. Wen Y, Feng P, Zhang H, et al. Comparison between allogeneic tendon fixation and screw fixation in ligamentous Lisfranc injury: a biomechanical analysis. Sichuan Da Xue Xue Bao Yi Xue Ban 2013;44:222–5, 41.
31. Nery C, Réssio C, Alloza JF. Subtle Lisfranc joint ligament lesions: surgical neoligamentplasty technique. Foot Ankle Clin 2012;17:407–16.
32. Buzzard BM, Briggs PJ. Surgical management of acute tarsometatarsal fracture dislocation in the adult. Clin Orthop Relat Res 1998;(353):125–33.
33. Hsu A, Moss L, Harris TG. Dorsal plating of low-energy Lisfranc injuries: a case report. Foot Ankle Spec 2015;8:73–6.
34. Stern RE, Assal M. Dorsal multiple plating without routine transarticular screws for fixation of Lisfranc injury. Orthopedics 2014;37:815–9.
35. Alberta FG, Aronow MS, Barrero M, et al. Ligamentous Lisfranc joint injuries: a biomechanical comparison of dorsal plate and transarticular screw fixation. Foot Ankle Int 2005;26:462–73.
36. Arntz CT, Veith RG, Hansen ST. Fractures and fracture-dislocations of the tarsometatarsal joint. J Bone Joint Surg Am 1988;70:173–81.
37. Trevino SG, Kodros S. Controversies in tarsometatarsal injuries. Orthop Clin North Am 1995;26:229–38.
38. Chiodo CP, Myerson MS. Developments and advances in the diagnosis and treatment of injuries to the tarsometatarsal joint. Orthop Clin North Am 2001;32:11–20.
39. Aitken AP, Poulson D. Dislocations of the tarsometatarsal joint. J Bone Joint Surg Am 1963;45-A:246–60.
40. Hirano T. Newly developed anatomical and functional ligament reconstruction for the Lisfranc joint fracture dislocations: a case report. Foot Ankle Surg 2014;20(3):221–3.

Index

Note: Page numbers of article titles are in **boldface** type.

Foot Ankle Clin N Am 21 (2016) 177–206
http://dx.doi.org/10.1016/S1083-7515(16)00009-7
1083-7515/16/$ – see front matter © 2016 Elsevier Inc. All rights reserved.

Moving?

Make sure your subscription moves with you!

To notify us of your new address, find your **Clinics Account Number** (located on your mailing label above your name), and contact customer service at:

Email: journalscustomerservice-usa@elsevier.com

800-654-2452 (subscribers in the U.S. & Canada)
314-447-8871 (subscribers outside of the U.S. & Canada)

Fax number: 314-447-8029

Elsevier Health Sciences Division
Subscription Customer Service
3251 Riverport Lane
Maryland Heights, MO 63043

*To ensure uninterrupted delivery of your subscription, please notify us at least 4 weeks in advance of move.

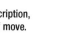

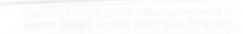

Printed and bound by CPI Group (UK) Ltd, Croydon, CR0 4YY

08/05/2025

01864682-0001